Dr Chavi Eve Karkowsky

high risk

a doctor's notes on pregnancy,
birth, and the unexpected

SCRIBE
Melbourne • London

Scribe Publications
2 John Street, Clerkenwell, London, WC1N 2ES, United Kingdom
18–20 Edward St, Brunswick, Victoria 3056, Australia

Published by Scribe 2020

High Risk is a work of nonfiction. All patient names and potentially identifying
details have been changed, along with the names and descriptions of certain
other individuals.

Book design by Ellen Cipriano
Printed and bound in the UK by CPI Group (UK) Ltd, Croydon CR0 4YY

Scribe Publications is committed to the sustainable use of natural resources and
the use of paper products made responsibly from
those resources.

9781913348083 (UK edition)
9781925849974 (Australian edition)
9781925938258 (e-book)

Catalogue records for this book are available from the National Library of
Australia and the British Library.

scribepublications.co.uk
scribepublications.com.au

Contents

TERM PREGNANCY

GOING INTO THE HOSPITAL
(OR STAYING OUT)

POSTPARTUM AND BEYOND

Introduction

No Little Thing

I met Yvonne Donaldson when she was 8 weeks pregnant. Her other doctors couldn't quite believe it: she was over 40 and had almost no working organs in her body. Her lifetime of severe diabetes and hypertension had left her with renal failure, heart failure, strokes, and a myriad of other diseases. She was on dialysis three times a week. And yet here we were, with a small flickering shape on the ultrasound.

I rarely counsel any patients toward termination if the pregnancy is desired. I recommend it only if I really, truly think that there is a high chance of the woman dying because of the pregnancy or delivery. But Yvonne's body was barely managing day-to-day function; a pregnancy was risky and delivery almost definitely life-threatening. Then there was the fetus: Yvonne was on multiple medications that were terrible for developing hearts and brains. Nobody had ever discussed changing them because none of her doctors seemed to have thought of her as someone who could become pregnant—as someone who had sex, who desired and was desired.

Now, with Yvonne 8 weeks pregnant, I had met her twice. I had met her husband and seen her older kids sitting in the waiting room. When I had finally gathered all the information that I could about her besieged body, I told her what I saw as the truth: the path to an actual live baby was narrow, and we might well lose her along the way. I recommended that she think seriously about termination of pregnancy in order to save her own life. She smiled at me, the way someone smiles who has been told she's going to die by many people for many years. "Dr. K., no offense. But ain't no little thing gonna happen."

After each hours-long session with her and with her family, answering questions, predicting bad outcomes, feeling that Yvonne didn't take me seriously, I would drag myself off to my office, drained and exhausted. I would say to my fellow doctors, "She's wrong. Because every little thing is going to happen. Every. Little. Thing."

As it turns out, we were both wrong. And we were both right.

. . .

SOMETIMES YOU KNOW you're going to need a maternal-fetal medicine doctor; you've always known. Perhaps you've had an autoimmune disease for years, or a heart condition, or a kidney transplant, and you knew that if you ever got pregnant, you would be "high risk." Maybe your last baby was born early or you've had multiple miscarriages and are finally ready to try again. In these cases, you know you are going to need a doctor like me, a maternal-fetal medicine specialist (also known as an MFM specialist, a perinatologist, or, more colloquially, a "high-risk pregnancy doctor"); we're obstetrician-gynecologists who have undergone further training to become specialists in maternal and fetal high-risk conditions. If we're really prepared, perhaps we even met with you long before you got pregnant and planned your medications and your management so that everything could be as healthy and calm as possible.

But often, that's not who you are. Often, you didn't know you were going to need us; you were completely, boringly healthy and having a completely, boringly routine pregnancy—until all of a sudden, you were not. Sometimes you're a 33-year-old having your second baby when an ultrasound finds something not quite right about the shape of the fetal heart. Sometimes your water breaks at 27 weeks despite having no risk factors and no warning. Sometimes you're a woman in a clinic who thought she just had a heart murmur, but the endurance event that is pregnancy reveals a complicated cardiac condition that makes carrying and delivering your pregnancy life-threatening. Sometimes you're a 19-year-old newly postpartum mom, bleeding too much too fast; now you are a high-risk pregnancy, after the birth, despite the low-risk status of everything up to this moment.

Taking care of any of that—of all of that—is my work.

.   .   .

I WROTE THIS book because I think I have the most interesting work in the world. When I decided to become a doctor, part of what I learned about myself—a heretofore mild, book-loving nerd—is that I am a bit of an adrenaline junkie. I thought I was going to be a psychiatrist or a pediatrician. I thought I would be someone who sat in a room with a clipboard: more talk, less action. But once I was involved in medicine, I was immediately addicted to the action (though I still love to talk). I wanted to be part of the muchness of it, the everyday drama and blood and terror and joy.

I think this muchness is appealing for a lot of high-acuity specialties—trauma surgery and emergency medicine are two other examples—anything where life and death things happen, and happen quickly. But I think I chose MFM because there is a way in which it is a field that has the most of this muchness. This is partially a result of the pace and volume of obstetrics, but also because it is a funny mix of routine (so much of the world has a baby, and everyone has been one) and awe (which even an uncomplicated delivery can provide).

As the name implies, maternal-fetal medicine is a specialty that deals with pregnancy, yes, and birth, and the medical and obstetric complications therein. But that's just the beginning of what we do. Our work includes the wide spectrum that is reproductive life: infertility, pregnancy loss, terminations of pregnancy, contraception. We are dealing with birth, but also death. We are dealing with the most private of parts of the body and sometimes the heart. We are dealing with the vulnerable, the beloved, the doted-upon, and the neglected. We are dealing with a life cycle event about which people have expectations in a way that they don't about appendectomies or MRIs. Wrapped up in that life cycle event are strong feelings about gender, sexuality, family, and almost every aspect of being human.

This work in high-risk pregnancy offers a window into the darkest and lightest corners of people's lives, into the extremes of human experience. I am honored to be with people through their worst tragedy, in their deepest shame, and during their greatest joys. Sometimes I get to walk with them from one to the other, from tragedy through shame to joy. Such work is a privilege and a gift.

Despite the fact that pregnancy itself is central to so many of our plotlines—the sweet end to the romantic comedy, the bitter secret in the Victorian mansion, the punchline in the sitcom—in my experience almost nobody knows what can happen during, before, or after a pregnancy. Nobody—not regular people, not all doctors, certainly not many of our policy makers—seems to understand what happens in our clinics and hospitals. In this work, I think I see the most interesting and subtle and extreme situations in the world; and I also see that most of the world knows almost nothing about it.

. . .

YVONNE GOT PREGNANT because none of her vast and experienced medical team, doctors she saw every day, ever addressed contraception or fertility. They never talked about this part of her health, of her body, of her life.

I think that Yvonne stayed pregnant in part because the way she thought about her body in pregnancy was different from the way she thought about it in every other circumstance. This pregnancy was something different for her: a family event, not a medical one; a spiritual event, not just a bodily one. It was, she told me, a miracle.

Yvonne was willing to take risks she would never otherwise consider. She was willing to lie down on the altar of illness for the idea of a baby, one that might never exist. Just like her many doctors, but for very different reasons, she didn't want to talk about her reproductive health.

. . .

I THINK THAT few people know what happens in this work because, culturally, in the media and in art, pregnancy is often shorthand for "happily ever after": no complication, nuance, or exploration. What the experience of reproductive life actually can mean to a woman, in all its bloody complexity, is almost never inspected in any real way in our art or media.

Here's what I've noticed: I'll go to a dinner party or a picnic, and I will be asked what I do for a living. Within 15 minutes, I will be ruining that dinner party or picnic because I'll be in the middle of a very intense conversation about epidurals or placentas or miscarriages: not the usual cocktail hour stuff. Sometimes I'll be having that conversation with a woman, but quite often with a man; sometimes with a father, but sometimes with an aunt or a grandfather or a sister-in-law. These will be people who, months or years after their experience of reproductive life, are still processing what happened to themselves or to someone they love, and finding it hard to do so. It may be wonder or joy that they're processing, but mixed in there is often a fair amount of fear and a nontrivial measure of anger.

Even if these individuals knew the facts—had read a pregnancy book or taken a hypnobirthing class—something about this reproductive life experience was new and wonderful or new and terrible. They're still adjusting to what happened because they were completely unprepared for much of what they saw or felt.

At that dinner party, we'll discuss the epidural administered too late or the cesarean delivery too early; the shabby clinic where they had to go for a termination or even just the repeated small embarrassments of the care they received. What they are grappling with, I think, is some measure of cognitive dissonance. There's the distance between the bodily truth of these experiences and what the rest of our curated lives has prepared us for. There is also, I think, surprise at the way that becoming a patient is such an immediate transition into powerlessness. There's a lot of emotional experience to unpack, but the most common phrase I probably hear is this: "I wish someone had told me."

This lack of nuance and depth is a problem for all medical fields, but I do think it's an especially difficult problem with respect to pregnancy and pregnancy complications. For one thing, as I've mentioned, we have expectations of pregnancy that we don't have of other medical experiences. We expect a pregnancy and its outcome to make us happy and to complete us; we don't have such expectations from an appendectomy or a bone density scan.

But I also think it's a problem because more of us are affected. Though it's true that we probably don't talk enough about the nuance in heart attacks or cancer, not everybody has a heart attack, and not everybody has cancer. But everybody is born.

In our larger public discussion, we don't talk about reproductive health and its possible complications, all it can involve, in any real or helpful way. We gloss, we elide; we buy pink and blue balloons, and we let the conversation end there. This lack of depth, it turns out, creates some big problems.

· · ·

AS HER PREGNANCY progressed, Yvonne got sicker and sicker. Her blood pressure became almost impossible to control; her sugar values were low, then high. Her dialysis was now 6 days a week in an effort to help clean her blood and give her pregnancy better odds, but those hours attached to a machine were taking their toll. Yvonne was 24 weeks pregnant when we admitted her to the hospital; ordinarily that would have been a fetus that could, if necessary, have a chance of surviving outside its mother. But this pregnancy had not grown well, largely due to Yvonne's extensive vascular disease. The uterus and placenta had the same problems as the rest of her body, and so the pregnancy was not well fed; her 24-weeker looked more like a 20-weeker. After long and complicated discussions with the neonatology team and Yvonne, we decided not to check on this baby too often. We couldn't deliver her; she wouldn't survive at that weight. We checked the fetal heart once a day, and Yvonne knew that any day we could look for a heartbeat and find none, a pregnancy that finally received too little oxygen or too few calories via its meager placenta to continue.

Then 25 weeks passed. Despite the difficulties of its in utero environment, there was always a fetal heartbeat. Then 26 weeks passed, then 27 weeks. At 28 weeks, the fetus finally measured 500 grams, close to what an average 24-weeker would weigh. Based on those long ongoing discussions with the pediatric team and the patient, we decided to start fetal testing on this compromised pregnancy.

On her first day on the fetal monitor, Yvonne's fetal tracing looked terrible; it was a pattern consistent with a fetus that was not getting enough oxygen. Nobody wanted this ill patient to end up in an emergency cesarean delivery, so we mobilized for a cesarean during the day, with all anesthesia, critical care, renal, and other teams ready to go.

Yvonne went to the operating room (OR). She went all the way to sleep because her heart function made it dangerous for her to get the usual spinal anesthesia. The team made a large vertical incision on her belly in order to give this baby the gentlest possible trip out. When they got to the uterus, they bivalved it open like an oyster shell; it hadn't grown enough to deliver the baby any other way. The baby was handed to the neonatology team, who put the smallest tube they had down her throat. They wheeled the baby to the neonatal intensive care unit (NICU); an hour later, my team wheeled our patient, also still asleep with a tube down her throat, to the adult ICU. We were not sure either of them would survive.

. . .

THE RUINING-COCKTAIL-PARTIES problem isn't just an individual dilemma. When our media representation of pregnancy stops at the uncomplicated and adorable, that gives us, as a society, a problem on multiple levels. As individuals, women are often left unprepared to make decisions or shaken after the fact, traumatized because the image they were given of pregnancy is just so very far from their lived truth.

The lack of real representation is also a problem for families. Our stories of pregnancy, terminations, infertility, birth, and loss are the origin stories of every family. They are usually the primary event that we did—or didn't—go through. The fact that we don't have accurate media representation of these experiences may mean that we lose access to our own family history and to an understanding of the emotional landscape of the people we love the most.

Then let's go to a level beyond the family: the absence of nuanced discussion of women's health is a problem for us within the medical world, as patients and as physicians. Once, when I was working, a woman delivered a baby and then went into cardiac arrest. The obstetrics team called a code—a hospital-wide signal for a code team of several doctors, with special supplies, to race to us to initiate resuscitation. The code team for the hospital couldn't find us; not a single one of them had ever been on labor and delivery before. They didn't know which elevators to take or what floor to go to. Once they found the entrance to labor and delivery, they were stymied by a locked door. The labor and delivery unit had a special security system, designed to ensure that no babies would be kidnapped. But as part of this system, the hospital administration had neglected to make sure that the code team had access to this part of the hospital. Because of those decisions, because of the institution-wide inattention toward our entire discipline, precious minutes were lost before resuscitation was initiated. (The team was eventually let in by a medical student who heard the pounding on the locked door and led them to the right location.)

This is just one of a million examples of the ways that patients lose out because women's health is segregated into its own universe. I could tell you a thousand stories of delays in patient care because the emergency room doctor didn't perform a gynecological examination on a bleeding patient because they "didn't feel comfortable," thus allowing her to hemorrhage longer in the ER. I could tell you a dozen more stories of neurosurgeons with whom I share the care of a patient with a small benign brain tumor; they cavalierly recommend a cesarean section because they think it will be easier on the patient (pro tip: it's not). Or I could tell you about the dialysis doctors who never thought to offer contraception to Yvonne or at the very least to send her to someone who could.

The costs of this silence don't end there. When we don't talk about women's health, our leaders and governments make policy about women's bodies every day with precious little accurate information. Much of the time, that policy is made by people who have no experience either inhabiting a body with female reproductive capacity or the knowledge of what it requires to care for one. This leads to bad and often dangerous policy.

Finally, there's my personal level: I'm an MFM specialist, and I've devoted my life to women's health. But I'm also a woman and a parent. To be perfectly honest, though I'm lucky enough to have gotten what I wanted out of my reproductive life, none of that journey was easy. I often found that the only people I could really talk to—the only people who understood what I was going through—were my colleagues. That didn't seem right. It seemed to me then and seems to me now that even people without MFM colleagues should have people who can understand what is happening, who have an understanding of this work.

This book is my way of bringing my work to you. Some of the stories in this book are mine; most of them belong to my patients. Before writing this book, I thought hard about the ethics of telling someone else's story. I struggled with multiple aspects of what it would mean to write this book: the inability to ask for permission to tell that story when these events were long ago, the need to protect patient confidentiality. My concerns were heightened because many of my patients come from underserved and routinely discriminated-against groups: women of color, women who live in some of the poorest neighborhoods in the United States. There is no question that they should have vastly more opportunities to tell their own stories. And, of course, there is the power differential inherent in our relationship: in most of these situations, I am the doctor; I am part of the institution that wields considerable influence over their bodies and lives. I am the one with the power. I am also, in these contexts, a white woman. This gives me another sort of power in many of my patient interactions. That's a level of privilege that I need to acknowledge.

In an attempt to address those differentials in privilege, I've made some choices throughout the book. Although all the stories in this book are true, I've used pseudonyms for all patients and changed identifying details to protect their anonymity. For the most part, I selected stories that happened years or even decades ago. In addition, the scenarios I bring to you happened more than once: I tell the story of a real patient, but the medical details of any case I use are clinical scenarios I've seen many times. Perhaps most importantly, I've tried to tell these stories with the realization that I am presenting my perspective and that I cannot know the whole story.

Even with those caveats, I decided to move forward and tell these stories; they are too important. In some ways, it is for those reasons—because I am a doctor, part of the system, the one with influence—that I hope people will start to discuss and acknowledge these stories. That is part of the power I have access to. By using this power to open this conversation, I hope that one day we will be able to bring forward the voices of the women who want to tell their own stories, in their own voices.

Throughout this book, I use the terms *women* and *females* to refer to female cisgender people. I do not mean to gloss over the existence of trans women or women without reproductive capacity for any reason. In addition, I know that trans men do get pregnant and have OBGYN needs and that those needs often go unmet, which is inexcusable. These people and their stories are compelling and important, and I'll read the hell out of a book on them. This book, however, is the stories of the patients I work with, a population almost exclusively composed of female cisgender people, and in this book I am generally using the language they use to refer to themselves.

Occasionally in this book, I'll tell a story and not tell you the ending. This has frustrated people: "But what happened?" they'll ask, sometimes with real anger. But the truth is that I don't always know the ending: the nature of my work is that people sometimes disappear. Sometimes the patients disappear: they get discharged or leave or just never come back to my clinic. Sometimes I'm the one who disappears: my in-service week is over or I move over to a new rotation or go on vacation or move to a new hospital. There will be stories without satisfying endings throughout this book because that's really how my work is; that's how life is.

This book is roughly organized in the order that we experience a pregnancy. However, it is not a guide through pregnancy, nor is it an exhaustive operator's guide for all the bad things that can go wrong for the owner of a uterus. This book may not, therefore, cover a particular issue or clinical situation; it may not cover important aspects of reproductive care, though it does cover a lot. Instead, this book is an exploration of the stories and patterns I've seen in my years in practice and in my own life, subject to the reflection that I think they deserve.

I wrote this book because my work grants me access to a corner of the world that is precious, beautiful, and hidden. That corner is universal and banal and everyday and by definition belongs to every single human. It's also full of extraordinary, once-in-a-lifetime, and complicated experiences that ask women and their families to be stronger, braver, and more vulnerable than most of us know. I wrote this book because women's health and reproductive health are human health; they are part of who we all are. I wrote this book because I think we need to see these stories and know them better.

. . .

Yvonne had a rocky course in the ICU; as we had feared, her management was a catch-22. She needed to be given fluid because without it her damaged heart did not pump very well; but when we gave her fluid, her lungs filled up with water because she had no functioning kidneys to filter and get rid of it. We had a roller coaster of dialysis and blood pressure control. Then there was concern for an infection and a possible clot in her leg. There were a couple of terrifying nights when it was all the ICU team could do to keep her vital signs close to normal range; there were a couple of nights when we weren't sure we would ever be able to wake her up.

But a few days later, things started to get better: Yvonne's breathing improved, and her breathing tube was removed. A week or so later, she came back to our pregnancy floor. A long while later, she was discharged to continue her dialysis and medical treatments from home.

She left long before her baby, who was one of the smallest in the NICU despite her relatively advanced gestational age. I used to see Yvonne being wheeled in to visit the baby. We would hug and exchange updates—Yvonne's heart was stable, but the baby's was worse; or Yvonne's sugar values were going crazy, but the baby's glucose was finally under control.

By the time Yvonne was discharged, the baby had all the complications of the extremely premature: breathing issues, nutritional challenges, infections. She had what looked like a possible stroke, and then on imaging of the head, moderate signs of brain damage, perhaps because of the stroke, perhaps because of the generalized stress of her in utero and ex utero life. The baby needed one surgery and then another. Four and half months later, the baby did eventually get discharged, alive. I don't know what her life has been like since then. I can't know what her life will be like in 10 years. I do know she's alive today, as I write this.

In the end, nothing out of the ordinary happened: a mother went home, and a baby went home, both alive. And yet, every little thing happened, and continues to, as it does every day.

FIRST TRIMESTER

1.

Nausea and Vomiting of Pregnancy

Did We Save Enough of Your Life?

Nausea is worse than pain.

I remember thinking this during the early days of my first pregnancy—a pregnancy I had prayed and wept for, despaired about, and agonized over. It was, as we say in obstetrics, a highly desired pregnancy. And yet, 6 weeks in, I found that I was hating every moment. Sometimes I would wake up and grab the sides of the bed, as if I were shipwrecked on an unstable raft. Lying there, my brain and stomach roiling, all I could manage was moaning; I couldn't try to roll over or sit up. There was something about the way my body existed in the world that was profoundly disorienting to my brain. Any movement made the disorientation worse, made my body reject what I was seeing. I wasn't immobile because of fear of vomiting, which offered awful and transient relief. I didn't move because I couldn't.

I remember calling my doctor's office after a day or two.

"Are you dehydrated?" the nurse practitioner asked. "Are you losing weight?"

"No. I don't think so. I mean, not yet. It's only been a couple of days," I said. "But I have clinic sessions tomorrow. I have to go to work."

She told me if I wasn't losing weight, I should try crystallized ginger. Maybe those acupressure bands for seasickness? But they didn't want to prescribe medications for nausea because they worried about the formation of the early fetus.

"But I have a job. I have to go to work. Just like you."

"You'll be fine, dear. Try the ginger."

I tried the ginger. I tried the acupressure bands. I tried vitamin B6. Nothing helped. I knew the medicines I was asking for weren't terribly risky; I had reviewed the data for my own patients and prescribed them many times. I also needed to get to work, to take care of those patients. Desperate, I wrote my own prescription for medications.

Once I got those medications into my body, I didn't feel great, or even good. But I was able to get up and get dressed. I was able to drive to my office. I was able to function and to sustain my livelihood.

. . .

NAUSEA AND VOMITING of pregnancy (NVP) is a common problem; it's so common—affecting 70 to 90 percent of pregnant women—that we sometimes have a hard time talking about whether it's a disease or just an unpleasantly normal part of what it means to be pregnant.

There are schools of thought that search for meaning in NVP. Did it once help pregnant women avoid toxins? It's unclear, though there's a lot of research invested in figuring it out. One of the most popular theories correlates the timing of NVP, the desire for bland foods, and a way to avoid foods that would cause harm to the fragile developing embryo during early pregnancy.[1]

We do know that there are correlations between NVP and decreased miscarriage risk, not because NVP makes pregnancies stronger, but actually the reverse: the hormones that the placenta produces are some of what is associated with the nausea, so a stronger, more effective placenta will be associated with more nausea. There are connections between thyroid disease and NVP, which may result from the fact that the thyroid hormone molecule and the pregnancy hormone human chorionic gonadotropin (the same one the urine stick tests for) have the same structure at one end and confuse the body; this is partly why NVP can look a lot like severe hyperthyroidism. Or maybe NVP happens because the stomach is more relaxed in pregnancy and has trouble emptying in a timely fashion.[2]

In the end, I find the search for a reason for NVP to be a distraction. It's pretty clear that however it started, and whyever it persists, the nausea that women experience in our current era doesn't help them or their pregnancy to be healthier or happier. In fact, it creates a situation in which some of the basic requirements of gestation— imbibing enough calories to grow a fetus; drinking enough water to allow an expanded blood volume to support a pregnant uterus— become difficult and sometimes impossible.

Giving the misery a reason, trying to find an evolutionary theory to make it meaningful, is very tempting; as humans we so often want or need to make meaning from the pain we experience. Arguably, we create a lot of art and beauty when we attempt to find that meaning.

However, just because the suffering can be made to make sense doesn't meant that it's necessary. Too often, the search for meaning in NVP comes at the cost of the main point: women are suffering. We can try to explain why NVP is important, evolutionarily; or we can narratively or theologically rely on misery being implicit in pregnancy and delivery ever since Eve partook of the fruit. All of these explanations start to make NVP seem valid or even necessary, a way that mothers must suffer for the miracle of gestation to make sense.

But of course, that's not true. Like many other physical sufferings, if NVP would magically disappear, that absence would harm no one. The eradication of the misery of NVP is a worthy goal. Sometimes the search for meaning obscures uselessness of the misery; it elevates the suffering at the cost of the sufferer.

That doesn't mean that there's no cost to treating NVP where our technology stands right now; there's always a cost, and there's always a limit to what medicine can do. As my nurse practitioner alluded to all those years ago, all maternal intake in the first trimester has a cost and a benefit. There's a price to the medications we take, often a price that we can't really know and may not know for years or decades. Sometimes the price is the un-knowing, the weightless shame that lands on us when we see our kid struggle with walking or need medication for ADHD or develop cancer. It probably wasn't related, right? That's what all the studies said. But we'll never really know, so the possibility often walks with parents forever as blame.

This is the main reason many women with NVP don't accept medication and why their providers don't offer it. Thankfully, for the vast majority of pregnant women, NVP is mild and transient without medications. However, even for these women, the experience can be difficult or even traumatic. When NVP is more severe, there can be higher prices to pay.

.   .   .

WE DO HAVE a name for severe NVP; when it crosses some invisible line, we call it hyperemesis gravidarum (HEG). That line is invisible because there are no clear criteria for starting to use the more severe label,[3] though it's pretty standard when the patient has intractable vomiting, clinical dehydration, and weight loss.

These days, I think of HEG as the darker side of NVP: the same product with the same packaging, but now with 20 percent more suffering and 60 percent more intractability. But before the age of reliable intravenous hydration or medications to capably combat nausea, HEG was more than that: it was potentially fatal.

Many cases of death from HEG occurred well into the early twentieth century and are described in the medical literature. The most famous death from HEG was probably Charlotte Brontë's (although whether or not her wasting disease was related to pregnancy is still controversial).[4]

The seriousness of HEG before the development of reliable IV hydration led to a lot of interest in treating the condition. Medical journals from the mid-nineteenth century discuss the wide use of bloodletting with leeches to offer relief from HEG; other options, such as purgatives or laudanum (an opiate), were also offered. One physician, writing in 1847, demonstrates the desperation of providers at that time by pointing out that "the mere enumeration of the various modes of treatment is a proof of the difficulty of combating the disease."[5]

If HEG would not resolve, faced with a patient with profound dehydration, malnutrition, and exhaustion, the physician would sometimes offer induction of "premature labor." Given the limited resources for premature babies or for neonatal resuscitation of any type, offering this treatment was really offering a termination of pregnancy (though some cases, described as term or near-term, did result in a surviving baby). This seems like an extreme measure to us now, as it did to them then. Fleetwood Churchill, in his 1847 textbook *The Diseases of Females*, finishes a technical discussion of how and why to induce labor in such patients by defending the practice ethically against naysayers:

> *It was now the middle of the seventh month, and I saw that she could not live till the ninth. I therefore proposed to bring on premature labour; but not liking to take the whole of the responsibility on myself, I desired the friends to send for some respectable person to meet me. The gentleman who came fell readily into my ideas, but did not see that the danger was so pressing. He therefore thought it better to wait for a fortnight longer . . .*
>
> [The patient worsens markedly.] *. . . I now told him, if he had not made up his mind, that I had. I added, that if he chose to undertake the bringing on of premature labour, he might: but I thought the time was past, and so did he. In two days more the patient sunk. Now I do not think it right to say that this woman would have recovered if premature labour had been brought on in proper time; but it is my opinion that it would.*[6]

Dr. Churchill ends by reinforcing what is at stake: "In such a case almost any remedy would be justifiable; and one that may afford an additional chance of safety to one of the parties implicated, must be hailed as a boon of great magnitude."[7] Desperate times called for medically desperate measures. In this case, success wasn't a healthy baby and a healthy mom; getting out of the pregnancy with the woman still alive was sometimes success enough.

In the 1800s, HEG wasn't considered merely bothersome; it wasn't treated as a figment of the imagination; it wasn't a subjective amorphous disease. It was common, real, and sometimes terrifying. Physicians took it seriously because this suffering was sharp, and it sometimes pierced all the way to pregnancy loss, death, or both.

. . .

SOMETIME IN THE early twentieth century, this attitude and approach changed. Intravenous hydration became available in the 1920s, and by 1945 it was commonplace for pregnant women.[8] After that, suffering from NVP and HEG was no less common, but it became far less common to die from it. Around that time, the way medicine started to think about these diseases changed a lot.

Part of what made NVP and HEG so confusing to nineteenth- and early twentieth-century science is that as the ability of medicine to diagnose conditions progressed, our understanding of these particular conditions was at a standstill. Autopsy studies of these patients, for example, would find, aside from the pregnancy, a complete absence of obvious structural reason for a woman to have suffered from this problem. There was no interesting pathology—no blockages, no anatomic malfunctions, no intestines turning colors, no colons blowing up like balloons. As the condition became less fatal but continued to be common, medicine left behind its anatomic tools and began to turn to the nonphysical to explain what was going on. Neurology was poorly understood, but the malfunction of the nervous system seemed a reasonable, invisible explanation for NVP and HEG; these diseases were then called, as was the style of the time, a kind of neurosis. When early psychiatry and Freud came along, the psychoanalytic thought and philosophy that were beginning to influence almost all aspects of science and culture folded beautifully into the neurotic explanation for the cause of HEG and NVP.

In 1881, F. Ahlfeld cured a patient of her HEG through entirely psychiatric treatment (during the very year that Freud graduated from medical school), and for decades, this case was cited as evidence of the psychiatric basis of the problem.[9] Freud's teachings were easily integrated into the understanding of neurosis as the cause of HEG, which was further attributed to "the abhorrence of the process of impregnation, the loathing of the husband, and of the expected child."[10] These ideas had tremendous staying power; a typical article from 1968 by Denys Fairweather introduces a discussion of NVP and HEG by saying that "in most of the severe cases, there are elements of underlying emotional disturbance."[11] The psychological rationale for HEG was offered to patients as late as the 1990s.[12] The psychiatric connection was so powerful and so long-lived that it was at least mentioned in almost all discussions of NVP or HEG throughout the twentieth century, so much so that the current guidelines of the American College of Obstetricians and Gynecologists (ACOG) still address the question: "Is there a role for psychotherapy in treatment [of NVP]?" (The answer, at least by 2004, was, "There is little evidence for a therapeutic effect.")[13]

Within the neurotic explanations of HEG, nuance did exist: the vomiting was described as any or all of the following: "a rejection of femininity or a rejection of pregnancy and impending motherhood via an unconscious, oral attempt at abortion."[14] Other schools of thought saw HEG as an ambivalence (rather than rejection) of pregnancy, with nausea and vomiting representing the inner conflict between wanting and rejecting the baby.[15] Other theories implicated sexual frigidity and relational immaturity,[16] thus relating the nausea not only to the pregnancy, but to the entirety of the woman's sexual and relationship history.

It is important to note that the neurotic theory of HEG never went unopposed. Doctors recalled the history of fatalities from HEG and reminded their colleagues that "no one dies from hysterics, and when a patient perishes from her disease, even if it greatly resembles hysterics, that is sufficient proof that it has not been hysterics."[17] A Dr. Ohlhausen wrote an editorial in 1904 reminding the medical world that "women suffering from hyperemesis are generally very sensible people."[18]

However, despite the voices of sensible doctors listening to sensible and miserable women, for decades the voices diagnosing psychotic and neurotic HEG were louder. During that time, those voices changed not just the perception of what caused the disease, but its treatment, and perhaps most importantly, how it felt to have the disease.

Through much of the twentieth century, treatment modalities for HEG tended to at least include some mention of psychotherapy, and analysis became a mainstay of treatment. This could have been benign, if not terribly effective, but other treatments started to cross the line from treating a physical ailment to addressing—or punishing—a mental one. Some examples include the recommendation that patients not be given a receptacle for vomit or be cleaned up, but be left to vomit in their bed, so that they could fully understand the ramifications of what was understood to be their choice. One doctor ordered patients to have no contact with their husbands or families in a treatment meant to address her antipathy toward them, which was—to their thinking—the underlying cause of the nausea. Other protocols encouraged the physician to invoke fear in order to counteract the neurosis that was supposedly behind the nausea to begin with.[19]

These tactics were never universally adopted and were often applied with whatever compassion or empathy could be mustered. However, when I look now at the application of the psychiatric explanation and resulting treatments of NVP, the total effect seems to be one of enormous amounts of anger directed at pregnant women suffering from the condition. Despite what were likely good intentions, by subscribing to a worldview where NVP and HEG were invented mental problems, both doctors and patients entered a universe where it was acceptable not only to dismiss women's suffering, but to blame them for it.

The suffering woman was not just blamed for her NVP and HEG, but worse, blamed for her developing relationship with motherhood, for her unsatisfying sexuality, and for the shortcomings of her marriage. In this universe, this patient, pregnant and miserable, is manifesting her failure as a wife, mother, and sexual partner—in effect, as a woman. Furthermore, within the thinking that represents HEG as a neurosis, she is also a liar, because if the woman says she wants to be pregnant but then is vomiting, her nausea is understood as the clear evidence of her real motives: her rejection of her progression to motherhood, her hatred of the men in her life, her dislike of the sexual act that the pregnancy represents, or all of the above.

If HEG at the time was considered a neurotic disease, then it makes sense that the treatments of that time seemed more interested in aligning the misery of the body with the presumed misery of the mind. Reduction of misery, the alleviation of suffering, had very little place in the definition of successful treatment.

Today, of course, we think we're relatively enlightened. And today, NVP and HEG still exist. In any hospital I've ever worked at, there are at least one or two HEG patients admitted in early pregnancy at any given time. (If they're sick enough to be admitted to the hospital, we usually are well within the parameters of the more severe diagnosis of HEG.)

. . .

I MET VICTORIA Crusan, a patient with terrible nausea in pregnancy, as I rounded on the patients on the high-risk pregnancy service during one of my weeks as the inpatient attending. Victoria was 21 years old and at the start of her first pregnancy; she had been admitted overnight. Victoria was about 8 weeks pregnant, according to the resident accompanying me who got me up to speed on the patient's history: like many patients with HEG, Victoria had been bouncing from emergency room to emergency room for a few weeks, with at least four visits in the last 10 days. Each time, she was given antiemetic medications and some IV fluids. Often, she improved enough to eat a cracker or sip some juice. With this evidence of cure, she was sent home. Once home, sometimes she would be able to fill the prescription she was given; sometimes it would be impossible because she was given a hard time by her insurance company or a pharmacist ("I think these medications aren't a great idea in pregnancy. You need to have your doctor call us before we can dispense these") and was having a rough time getting out for even the short trips those errands required. Even when she managed to get the pills, Victoria was almost never able to keep them down once she swallowed them.

Within 12 hours of her discharge, she'd start vomiting again, spend the next day becoming dehydrated again, and go around this nightmarish merry-go-round again. At the time of my visit, her first morning in the hospital, it had been at least 2 weeks since she'd had any sort of real nutrition or anything approximating the caloric intake that humans need to survive.

Last night, someone finally noticed how dehydrated and malnourished Victoria looked, how it was her second visit at our same emergency room; that there was a pattern here that a cracker and some juice were not going to break. The decision was made to keep her in the hospital, at least overnight.

This morning, when we walk into Victoria's room, it's dark even though it's past 10 am. The curtains are drawn in the dim room, and it smells terrible, though I know she came up from the emergency department only about 8 hours ago. This is pretty typical for HEG patients; Victoria's been feeling terrible for weeks and probably hasn't slept much, so she's always exhausted. Her caloric deficit and constant nausea make hygiene really challenging; even when she's not throwing up, she seldom has the energy to bathe.

In the dark room, Victoria is immobile and wrapped in a mountain of blankets. She's cold because her body has been essentially starving since this pregnancy started. For a moment, as we walk in from the brightness of the hallway, I can't find Victoria, her body so still, another lump among the piles of bedding. She is on her way to disappearing, literally and figuratively eaten by her own pregnancy.

Once the decision was made to admit Victoria to our inpatient service, Victoria started receiving medications and treatments designed to help her. The medications we use include ones that were explicitly invented to treat nausea, but others started life as anti-seizure drugs or antianxiety drugs, with their incidental side effect now the main benefit. As with many diseases in pregnancy, we end up using the oldest drugs. They're often not the most effective or even the least toxic medications for nausea, but because they're old, they're always the ones with the most years of reports about birth defects and other pregnancy-associated risks. Because it's so ethically fraught and difficult to do research on pregnant women, pregnant women end up with subpar options in this way, but we do what we can, as safely as we can.

Most HEG patients need more than one medication to make any sort of progress toward their normal life, and so despite the fact that we'd like to minimize risks to the fetus, I often need to recommend adding a second or a third so that we can make progress toward having Victoria eat enough to support her body and a growing pregnancy.

This morning, as I meet her and ask to feel her stomach, I try to talk to Victoria about adding a new medication, about the risks and benefits. I also want to make sure this pregnancy is desired and that she wants to continue it; I want to find out more of what's going on in Victoria's life and what kind of damage her illness has done to it. But Victoria is not interested in talking or listening much. She nods to allow me to do a quick abdominal exam and sits up a little bit. She answers my question of whether this is a desired pregnancy with a soft but clear "yes." But she never completely opens her eyes, and after a sentence or two, she shakes her head and slides back down under her covers, gone again.

As we walk out of Victoria's room, I review the plan I've made

with the resident. This morning we are trying Victoria on medications through the IV, but later today we'll try to switch her to a medication that can be absorbed from the inside of her cheek; and when
she gets a little better, we will encourage her to learn how to give herself rectal suppositories. These are all ways to actually get the medicine into her body when she doesn't have access to an IV, because
asking a vomiting woman to get an antinausea pill to stay down long
enough to work can be an exercise in futility. The more options she
has at home, the more likely she'll be able to stay there.

For right now, Victoria is also getting vitamins and sugar
through the IV. In the short term, these substances can prevent
some of the worst complications of dehydration and malnutrition.
But we can't give real nutrition—protein, fats—through the IV line,
so even with our interventions, she continues to starve. The plan
is to get her to the point that she can tolerate oral intake and feed
her body through her mouth. We can try that once her stomach has
really had a chance to rest—perhaps tomorrow morning if our current medication regimen is successful.

But if Victoria does not improve and become able to take in real
nutrition orally within a few days, we'll have to talk about even more
invasive measures. We can try to put a tube in her nose, down her
throat, into her stomach to treat her. This option is appealing only
because the alternative is worse; we can put a long-term, large catheter in her vein to be able to give her nutrition, but those catheters
and the associated feeding is well known to be rife with severe complications: clots and hard-to-treat infections.

We'll also ask our mental health team to see Victoria. She may
be depressed, but she also may just be miserable. Many of the studies supporting a psychiatric foundation for HEG confirmed that

depression is more common in women who suffer from nausea in pregnancy. Of course, this is a classic example of flawed study design, creating research to confirm your own assumptions. Were these women nauseous because they were depressed? Or were they depressed because of their debilitating nausea?

Even when Victoria is off of IV medications and eating a bit of actual nutrition, she might stay a day or two more as an inpatient. Most of these HEG patients have already bounced around the system, and that's in large part because this particular diagnosis is usually marked by repeat discharges and readmissions. A lot of what she needs to keep her out of the hospital isn't medical but logistical: a relationship with a pharmacy, stable health insurance, a clinic that can see her quickly if she gets worse. Discharge planning like this takes time but can pay back in reduced hospitalizations and, we hope, reduced misery.

The most important part of our treatment plan has less to do with Victoria's body and more to do with her state of mind. Later today, after Victoria's had some more sleep and a few hours without vomiting, we'll air out her room. The nurses will offer to help her shower. Victoria will talk with our social worker, who agrees that Victoria isn't depressed, just miserable.

Once her nausea is somewhat treated, she reverts to her usual personality, though she is still clearly struggling with the burden of feeling unwell. Once that's done, I'll be able to come back and sit on the side of her bed and say, "We need to talk about what we can accomplish, and how much 'better' is enough."

HEG is supposed to be a first-trimester disease; it's supposed to improve and remit as hormone levels stabilize after 14 weeks. Often it does, but sometimes it doesn't. The secret to a successful pregnancy with HEG is the setting of appropriate expectations and the structure of self-care in what may be challenging weeks or even months.

Sitting on the side of Victoria's bed, we will talk. "I hate to say this," I will say, "but even with all our medications and gadgets and tricks of the trade, we may not get you all the way back to your old self. Even if we do, it may take a few weeks or even longer. I hope that's not true, but we need to figure out what we can get to, what we will call success. And what your life will look like during that time." Victoria will not be able to go back to her old life right now. She may be able to go back to work with a careful medication regimen; her semester at school may be salvageable. But she may not be able to function at either of those places, and we will need to plan for that, too.

In the end, Victoria will stay with us for almost a week, feeling a bit better every day. She is eventually discharged home with literal sacks of medications; we will bargain with the hospital pharmacy to fill all her prescriptions before she leaves so she'll have one less reason to be back. We discharge her, and we wave as she walks out with her boyfriend. Later that week, we notice that she hasn't been back to the emergency department. We did a good job, right? That's success, isn't it?

· · ·

VICTORIA'S CASE WAS severe, but even less serious cases of NVP are traumatic. I have one friend, Andrea, whose nausea during her two pregnancies had been, by formal criteria, mild. Always slender, she lost only a bit of weight during her pregnancies; she never required hospitalization or even an emergency department visit for IV hydration. There's no entry in the clinical record for "I routinely had to leave the class I was teaching to throw up behind a sofa and then go back to finish the class" or "I could so rarely focus on my lab projects that my tenure was delayed by at least a semester." Her medical record of that time looks unremarkable. If you ask her doctors, they would probably say that her pregnancy had some early mild NVP but was otherwise uncomplicated. In many important ways, it was: healthy mom, healthy baby.

But three years after her second birth, Andrea was diagnosed with cancer. She had young children, a loving husband, and a great career. Andrea had every reason to be aggressive with her chemotherapy. And yet, she told me, when her doctor sat down to present her with a treatment plan, she stopped him and told him, "I can't do it again. I can't go through that nausea again." Her first order of business, when facing the treatments that could save her life, was to extract a promise from her oncologist that she would never, ever feel like she did during her pregnancies. Her nausea was so horrible a memory that she couldn't even consider taking on chemotherapy until this concern was addressed.

On paper, in her medical chart, Andrea had an uncomplicated pregnancy, but I think if you asked Andrea her own recounting of that time, she'd tell you that it was the hardest time in her life up to that point. Years later, the memory of that time, the suffering she went through, needed to be addressed before she would even begin discussing something as serious as her cancer treatment. That suffering was never really dealt with during her pregnancy, or even noted.

Was her NVP really mild? Were her pregnancies really uncomplicated?

How successful, in the end, was her success story?

. . .

LONG AGO, WOMEN used to die from NVP and HEG. During that
time, the desperation of their doctors was apparent; without effective treatment or nutritional support, the medical establishment was
grateful to get any patient out alive, a truly elemental definition of
success. One day, women stopped dying from these diseases, and
when they did, we physicians lost our desperation. At around that
time, NVP became a disease of the mind. Within that setting, successful treatment of NVP was more about making women face that
lie than relief from suffering; in fact, sometimes increasing the suffering was part of the treatment.

No qualified medical professional believes that NVP is in the
patient's mind anymore. Today, no legitimate doctor or midwife
would tell a patient with NVP that she is frigid or that she secretly
wants to abort her pregnancy. Still, the misery persists, and still our
definition of success is inadequate.

Sometimes the misery persists because, as in my first pregnancy,
the medical establishment still doesn't value the suffering of the
mother over the smallest possible risk to her growing fetus. I wasn't
about to die or require hospitalization, so nobody asked me if that
was successful enough. I was losing function; I was losing my livelihood and a large part of what makes life fulfilling to me. But nobody
asked me.

Sometimes the misery persists because, as with Andrea, the
medical establishment doesn't even see that we still have a problem,
that HEG still causes suffering on a par with diagnoses like cancer that carry a more serious attentiveness from the medical field.
Nobody asked Andrea if she was better enough, if her nausea treat-

ment was successful; her reaction, years later, tells us that the answer was a very clear no.

And sometimes the misery persists, as for Victoria, because although no qualified modern provider will tell a woman it's all in her mind, nobody bothers to look at her larger life. In every emergency department visit, modern medicine was used to keep Victoria alive—success for that day, for that hour. She received IV fluid; she ate a cracker. But for weeks Victoria bounced in and out with no doctor assessing the larger picture. Nobody noticed her weight plummeting or that she hadn't eaten protein in several weeks; if they noticed, they didn't do anything about it. Not their problem—they kept her alive for that day, they did their job.

Sometimes you can judge medical success by numbers: Did the cholesterol go down or the blood pressure go up? Did the pregnancy complete at least 37 but no more than 42 weeks of gestation? Was the newborn weight at least 2,500 grams? Did the patient die? Many of the successes we care about can be measured in those binaries. These answers can be averaged and logistically regressed and entered in a spreadsheet; they are easy to measure and to handle. The medical establishment loves these kinds of results for these very reasons.

But for other successes, the definition should be more complicated: did you decrease the suffering of the human before you? Part of what makes this success hard is that nobody can know the answer without asking that human who is before you, right now, what she thinks and what she wants and what she feels. Nobody asks, "Did we save enough of your life?"

If you don't ask her, the record will note "mild nausea, uncomplicated pregnancy," and nobody will note that she will always remember this as the worst time of her life. The record will note "multiple hospitalizations" but won't note "she finished the semester goddammit and graduated on time." You will miss the point of it all, almost all of the time.

. . .

VICTORIA ENDS UP transferring her prenatal care to our clinic, so I see her every few weeks for the rest of her pregnancy. We make sure she has access to meds, frequently assess her nausea, and tweak her medications. Even so, for the next month she ends up spending the night in the emergency department to get IV fluids and IV medications at least once every 10 days or so. But she never requires readmission, and we never end up having to place a permanent IV line. With the help of nutrition consult and fierce attention to what she can and can't tolerate, at 16 weeks she figures out what will and won't stay down—icy milkshakes end up being the key—and manages to stop her weight loss. We choreograph an elaborate network of inpatient and outpatient care to keep her out of the hospital, to keep her from getting dehydrated, to keep her from dying. We give her as much medicine as we know how; we are creative in the ways we give it. In turn, Victoria learns to show up at the clinic if nobody answers the phone; she learns how to make sure the doctors see her even if the appointment system can't figure it out.

Victoria never gains weight, but her belly grows nonetheless. Sometime after 26 weeks, the vomiting abates somewhat. I see Victoria in the clinic at 32 weeks; she is still profoundly nauseated and can't go back to work or school, but she has cut down to two medications and hasn't needed an emergency room visit for over a month. When we talk about this, I tell her that she should be really proud of herself—this has been tough to manage. It's been a full-time job—an unpaid, physically demanding, 24/7 unpaid job. Victoria manages a smile, but she has dark circles under her eyes, and when she gets up to walk down the hallway to make her next appointment, she is moving slowly, like a woman four times her age.

Victoria continues to feel nauseated until 39 weeks, when her water breaks. She goes into spontaneous labor and has an uncomplicated delivery.

Six weeks postpartum, I see her at a postpartum visit and don't recognize her. Today, she's an impeccably groomed young woman, a woman I would swear to you I have never seen before. She's wearing a silky shirt but really, it's her that's glowing; she is emitting light in my small exam room. A chubby baby girl is fitfully asleep in the stroller by the side of her chair. After the exam, as she's getting ready to go, she says, "Doctor, that was so terrible. That was the worst thing I've ever gone through. But I feel so much better now."

I've never asked her whether our care was good enough or whether her suffering was alleviated. I've never asked her if our treatment was successful, if we saved enough of her life. We worked so hard, and we gave her everything we had, and if I was honest, I don't think I can bear her answer. I don't ask her now.

"I'm so glad you feel better," I say, and she walks out to the rest of her life.

2.

Choosing a Provider

Scut Is Love

Here's a version of the party game "Would you rather?" Would you rather have a doctor who's kind and warm or a doctor who's good at her job?

I know that many people would say this is a false question. A doctor can be both, they would say. In fact, they would say that if a doctor isn't warm, kind, and accepting, then that doctor is not going to be as good at her job because she isn't listening and won't hear what she needs to know in order to be good.

But that's only sometimes true. Sometimes, in the depths of the repetitive, thoughtless tasks that make up much of a doctor's work, I have learned this: sometimes, when I'm a kind doctor, I'm farther from being a good one.

. . .

BY MY ABSOLUTELY invented calculations, 90 percent of the care that doctors provide has nothing to do with the job that medical school trained us for. About 10 percent of the job is deciding what medicine to give or whether surgery is advisable or performing the surgery; that's what they teach you in medical training. But the 90 percent that nobody teaches you is other stuff: documentation, filling out forms, renewing prescriptions, making phone calls so the surgical coordinator/visiting nurse service/pharmacy gets it right. It's dumb, inefficient, entirely necessary work, without which the surgery you performed, the medication you thought about, the plan you worked so hard on will just not happen. And that 90 percent of work is called, in medical parlance, "scut."

I don't remember this, but one of my friends told me that when she was an intern, demoralized by the hours and pages of scut before her, we had a talk. I told her that the scut was unbearably stupid and repetitive and beneath her and her decades of education. But scut was also how her patient was going to be able to leave the hospital and go home to her toddler or partner or job. Scut is paperwork, I apparently said, but scut is also love.

"Scut is love" is a motto for what I see as an important emotion for those of us who practice medicine, something I call pragmatic compassion. Pragmatic compassion is a particular form of sympathy or empathy, but what makes it powerful within medicine is both how necessary it is and how action oriented. Pragmatic compassion is how all that scut gets done, but more importantly, it's *why* all the scut gets done.

In your nonmedical life, it's the lady who stopped by unasked on the day a family member died, hugged no one, but dropped off a casserole. It's the mechanic who was condescending about a customer's gen-

eral lack of knowledge regarding outflow valves but saw the screaming
kid in the backseat and got the car on the road in record time.

Here's a small example: my 11 a.m. patient yesterday only spoke
Bengali. The basic professionalism drilled into me by my training
means that the visit will be competent. But the truth of our reality is
that any sort of productive and meaningful visit will require a boat-
load of pragmatic compassion. I need the pragmatic compassion so
that when I use the translator, which makes the visit three times as
long (doctor → translator → patient; patient → translator → doctor, at
the very least in the most straightforward of translational scenarios,
which happen approximately never), I don't lose patience. Pragmatic
compassion allows me, after covering the basics of the visit, to take
a few Bengali-English moments to make sure she has a childcare
plan for her young child when she goes into labor; this is not, strictly
speaking, my job, but I want to make sure that she understands what
she needs to do, so far from family and things she knows. Those
15 minutes won't figure largely in my notes; I can't bill for them.
But they're important, so I spend them. Arguably, none of the rest
of what I do—refilling her prenatal vitamins, managing her blood
pressure so that she stays safe, giving her a flu vaccine—is worth
much if she can't get to the hospital when she needs to.

I want to be clear that what I'm talking about isn't being "nice." I
wasn't particularly warm during this conversation (in fact, arguably,
my tone was irrelevant; the voice of the male translator may have
been the primary experience for this patient), because I was businesslike, running behind for other patients and in all likelihood a bit
harried. But we spent that 15 minutes, doctor → translator → patient;
patient → translator → doctor, because it's what she needed. That's
pragmatic compassion.

Compassion without pragmatism is inadequate because, in this work, we all learn early that "nice" has limitations. I learned this as an intern, when, in the spirit of egalitarianism and feminism, I tried to introduce myself on the labor and delivery (L&D) floor as Chavi. Not Dr. Karkowsky, no, no, no. Weren't we all care providers, all equal, all here for the same grand reason? The L&D nurses kicked that concept to the curb as soon as they heard it. For them, titles were not about higher or lower or medical school. Titles came down to something simple: what is your function? Can you write an order for a diet? Can you get me the medication I need for a patient? Because if you're a doctor, then you're a tool they know how to use and relate to. If you're Chavi, what exactly is your utility here? My attempts at "nice" hit a wall. Chavi was nice but useless; she had to go. Dr. K., now *she* could work.

Pragmatism without compassion is limited as well; in fact, compassion, in my experience, is not optional. Without some underlying regard or love for your patients, that effort, no matter how well meant, is just work, and for most humans, work without love hits a wall early. I am honored to have the most transcendent work, but even some of the most sacred work—delivering a baby, ushering a mother and baby safely through delivery—can, under the wrong circumstances, just become another draining source of exhaustion. As humans in a real world, with pain and terrible decisions, anger and 2 a.m. lab errors, we are often less than transcendent. Without the compassion, the work becomes difficult to enjoy, and quickly after that, almost impossible to do. The way forward, at 2 a.m., amidst blood and shit and amniotic fluid, is that potent fuel of pragmatic compassion. Scut is love, I think, because love is the only way to get the scut done.

Most of the time, pragmatic compassion is based on a narrative about the patient: "She's a single mom; I imagine it's hard for her to get to all of her ultrasounds"; or "the public transportation around here is awful; that's why she's always late to our appointments." Sometimes the narrative we have access to comes from the patient and is based on fact; however, often we invent one that makes this work easier. We tell ourselves a story in which this work is important and the recipient deserving; in that story, we can do the work because we need to. Thus, my friend managed the scut of discharge summaries when I manufactured a toddler (or partner or ailing parent or job) for her patient to go home to. And perhaps I spent time with the Bengali patient in part because I could pretend to understand the loneliness of the immigrant experience from my grandparents and of the worry of late pregnancy from my own.

In the end, that is the downfall of pragmatic compassion. It can be strong when the narrative is strong; but when the narrative fails, so can the compassion. Like many forms of kindness, it turns out that pragmatic compassion is easily broken.

Years ago, I was taking care of a 17-year-old patient with a really worrisome heart problem who kept missing appointments. Cardiology appointments were hard to come by, and office staff didn't always understand that pregnant patients can't wait six months until the next available appointment. I could have sent the patient to the front desk to try her luck with the appointment secretary; I could have sent her to the social worker and handed her off as a pregnant adolescent, please fix. Both of those options were available and technically appropriate. Both those options would have almost definitely ended up with an appointment long after her due date.

I didn't do that. I liked her. I liked her pink spiked hair and her terrible puns; I liked how she was trying to finish 11th grade, and I liked her overwhelmed and loving mom. I rode that like, and its accompanying pragmatic compassion, toward making four phone calls and e-mailing three providers, begging them to see this teenage patient before the month was out. When I gave her the appointment information, I told the patient that I had sold my firstborn two or three times just to get her that slot. Pragmatic compassion was how I got her a cab voucher so that there would be no barrier to her transportation to or from the appointment, and pragmatic compassion is how I called her the morning before to remind her of her appointment.

But my pragmatic compassion was also limited. Because the next day, she missed her appointment. When I called her to find out why, like any teenager she wouldn't pick up the phone. I ended up calling her mom and finally reaching my patient. "Why didn't you go? Why?" I got back only a sullen "I was tired, okay? I didn't want to wake up so early." There, right in the middle of that phone conversation, in my brightly lit office where I stole 2 minutes between patients to call her, I was tired, too, tired of this lazy kid. I felt the pragmatic compassion cracking off of me; I heard it falling away, hitting the floor so hard that it shattered on the tiles. I said something short and professional to her and got off the phone. I could have gotten on the computer right then and worked some magic; I could have wheeled and dealed to get her another appointment. I could have, but maybe I wouldn't. Maybe now I'd just send it to the secretary. Nobody could say I hadn't tried. Her scrappy teenage narrative was gone; and without it, I didn't really have the energy to do the extra work.

Here's another example. In a usual week, I field about 10 e-mails from the emergency department for an "urgent" new obstetric

appointment for a patient. One of our typical requests was for a
patient at 34 weeks gestation, newly arrived from India. This isn't an
unusual situation, and our clinics, ever aware of the ticking clock of
pregnancy, always try to get these patients into care as soon as possible. I ended up fitting in some extra time at the office and seeing this
patient myself at an ultrasound appointment. When she arrived, she
was nicely dressed. She spoke beautiful, accented English. She had
a new iPhone, much newer than mine, with all her records from
India on an app. I asked her why she had traveled so late in the pregnancy, and she said, "For a wedding. Vacation." For vacation? For a
wedding? For this reason I am now working late and adding her to
overbooked schedules and booting other patients who needed the
appointment—for vacation? The story that let me do extra work to
take care of her was a lie. And I had nothing underneath it.

I want to be clear: I did not commit malpractice. In the absence
of pragmatic compassion, I still finished her appointment. I still performed the physical exam; I still ordered labs; I still wrote my notes.
I wasn't rude; to the patient, the visit may have felt different, but
it was fine. Professional, Competent. Externally, the difference may
have been slight; I hope it was.

When the narrative collapses, does this make me less good at
that work? Even in my frustration, I know that the answer is probably yes. Subtly, finely yes, but yes. I've relied too much on pragmatic
compassion; when it fails, I am left without the compassion and with
just the dregs of the pragmatism. But this is the inevitability of the
world we live in and the humans we are: eventually, patients will fail
me, and if pragmatic compassion is all I have, then I will fail them.

This failure is in all likelihood because the narrative many of us
use to generate pragmatic compassion is too often predicated on a

form of paternalism. For this motivation to work, it seems that the doctor has to be the white knight, the patient the maiden in distress. This construction works only for such a narrow bandwidth of story that it too often doesn't work; it doesn't tolerate most of the truth that comes from working with fallible humans in a real world. If I want to function, something more solid needs to lie underneath. Something deeper and more unbreakable. Something that doesn't depend on a story or a feeling or a fiction. Something that is not about me or how deserving the patient is or how appealing the work.

You know how every time an abortion law comes up in the Supreme Court or in Congress, the airwaves are consumed by women who went through heart-wrenching choices? "I terminated my fetus," she wept, "because it wouldn't have lived." Or "I terminated my 20-week fetus," she cried, "because otherwise I would die."

These cases are true, and they happen every day, and they're a large reason why legal abortion is an important part of women's health care. But these stories are not the whole truth, because, it turns out, once termination of pregnancy is a legal and medical procedure, then it's a legal and medical procedure. When someone comes to the clinic to end their pregnancy, they are not asked if they've suffered quite enough to legitimate this procedure. They may be asked if they're certain; they should be asked if anyone has pressured them into this decision.

But for most routine terminations, nobody does the special arithmetic of misery: this much suffering + this much anguish = acceptable to perform the procedure. Termination of pregnancy, most days, is a medical procedure, so the patient either does meet the criteria or she doesn't. If she does, the doctor performs a technically competent procedure with appropriate interpersonal interaction. That's that.

This is hard for many people to believe, but the doctor performing the termination won't necessarily know that the patient already has two disabled kids and a partner who beat her and her kids until she ran away to a shelter (though this is too often the case); and the doctor won't know if, instead, the patient just doesn't want to be pregnant. Maybe it's even a terrible motivation; maybe the patient wants a boy, and testing has shown that this pregnancy is a girl, so she's terminating. Does the doctor not perform the procedure?

For most doctors, for whom the fetus is not a person and the patient most definitely is, the motivation of the patient, whatever the procedure, is not really relevant. The patient is an adult human who needs something. She needs a procedure, or she needs a first prenatal visit, or she needs a cardiologist. That's all, really, that needs to be known, and once that assessment is made, the path forward is clear.

That's not pragmatic compassion; that's professionalism, or even something less laudable, something closer to stubbornness. Whatever it is, it's reliable, and it will get you through the day when compassion has floated away and cannot be found again.

I once asked a friend, a provider of pregnancy terminations and one of the most dedicated physicians I know, whether she ever felt that a patient just didn't have reasonable justification for ending the pregnancy and what that cost her when it happened. My friend shrugged: "Most of our patients have really, really hard lives; that's usually why they're making a really hard choice. But even if they're not, even if this choice isn't hard for them—that's not really my business. I don't know her life; I'm not going to pretend I can."

That distance from the patient—"I don't know her life"—is ultimately, I think, the key. Pragmatic compassion depends on using your understanding of the patient—real, invented, sympathetic, empathetic, all or none of the above. Beyond that, and maybe purer than that, is "I don't know her life," which I'll term "compassionate distance." It sounds cold, but the cold is what gives it strength. It doesn't need your feelings to work properly; it stands alone, and because of that, it can't be broken. Compassionate distance is the humility to acknowledge that you can't, and maybe shouldn't, pretend to know what your patient is feeling, thinking, or choosing. She is an adult; she is human. You don't know her life. Isn't that enough?

An extreme example of this happens when trauma victims are brought into an emergency room. Trauma triage should, according to most medical ethicists, proceed without regard to crime or fault. So the shooter gets triaged just as the gunshot victim does; the drunk driver the same as the sober passenger. The more seriously injured one is the first to get a slot in the operating room without regard to moral deservedness.

For most bioethicists, this principle applies more painfully after a terrorist attack, when emergency departments are overwhelmed by bleeding and broken patients. Even then, even when all this pain and suffering was caused intentionally by one patient among many, the ethics of medical triage generally tell the providers to evaluate the patient in the suicide bomber vest by that patient's injuries, nothing more.[1]

Some of this guidance is rooted in the haste required by these terrible events: if we make the wrong judgment, if we mistake identity, we can't go back and prevent the innocent soul from bleeding to death. Are we ready to sentence someone to death based on the chaos that comes out of a bloody scene? That is a form of compassionate distance: our job that day is to provide medical care to the best of our abilities. The guilty and the innocent will be decided later, in court. Justice is, and should be, complicated, thoughtful, and slow. Today, I don't sentence anyone to death. Today, I don't know their life; let me save it, and then we will have the time to see.

For me, practice without pragmatic compassion is never going to be completely possible or even desirable. I need a little bit of warmth; I need the buzz of feeling like a good soul, of giving some affection and receiving it in return. I need the scut to be love.

I used to think that made me a better doctor—warmer, less robotic, the kind of doctor you'd want to find by your bedside during a terrible event or a tough delivery. But now I'm not sure that my reliance on pragmatic compassion doesn't make me a weaker one. My warmth is so fallible, my compassion so flawed.

I would rather be the kind doctor; it's much more pleasant. And I'm never going to give that up. But as it turns out, being a nice doctor is for me as much as it is for anyone else; it is, in some important ways, selfish and fallible.

So which would you rather have, a doctor who's kind and warm or a doctor who's good at her job? The better doctor—the doctor my patients should pick—is the one who doesn't rely on kindness to be good at her job, the one who knows that she can't know your life. She might not be warm, but that doctor? Her commitment is unbreakable.

3.

Genetic Testing

Everything Is Probably Okay

At the start of any first prenatal visit, I generally do an informal abdominal ultrasound. I warn the patient that it's a quick-and-ugly study; I get grainy images because I use the ultrasound machine that lives in my clinic, which is older than a lot of my patients. It works well enough to help me confirm the age of the pregnancy and the location within the uterus. But really, I perform the ultrasound so that we can see that first breathtaking flicker of a fetal heart.

What we are seeing is not always obvious to the patient or her partner. I generally spend a moment pointing out the outline of the uterus, the black universe of amniotic fluid surrounding the fetus, the fetus itself, and then finally the small pixelated area that pulses with a heartbeat. I point to it: "See how fast that's moving? That's the fetal heart, moving faster than yours. Much faster, like a humming-bird." Then I stop talking. It is almost always a moment of silence. It's not unusual for someone to cry.

Afterward, the patient wipes the gel off her stomach. Sometimes I offer her a hand to sit up. She takes a moment to rearrange her shirt, cover her belly, and swing her legs around the side of the table.

Then I sit down across from her and begin to soberly review an array of available genetic testing for various disfiguring and disturbing problems. I use words like "intellectual disability." I talk about Down syndrome, and I mention other, more severe diagnoses. I briefly mention pregnancy termination.

Right after the ultrasound, the patient is happy. She'd probably like to stay that way. And it would be so much easier to leave her happy. But that's not good medicine; and furthermore, it's not respecting her autonomy and her status as an adult with agency. So I lean forward and continue, because the twenty-first century has extremely powerful tools available for a woman to find out about possible problems with her pregnancy, and she deserves to know about them.

This is how I am professionally compelled to shatter the lovely ultrasound moment of joy and reassurance. This abrupt U-turn is hard to make without causing whiplash; and it can be traumatic, no matter how gently I try to do it.

In this first visit, I am trying to offer the patient information about prenatal diagnosis and the power over her own body and future that comes with it. But often, what she perceives is not information or empowerment or helpfulness; too often, what I've ended up providing is confusion, futility, or sometimes even complete betrayal.

·　·　·

PRENATAL TESTING CAN be unsettling in other ways. When we as a society test for a condition, what are we saying about the value of the lives of the people who have that condition? Prenatal testing shares some history with the eugenics movement, and though it is used differently now, it can provoke uncomfortable and important legal and ethical questions about disability rights. However, prenatal testing today—at least as it is supposed to be performed—is a different process, one focused on patient autonomy: on giving people information without direction as to how to use that information.

Prenatal diagnostic testing, particularly for genetic problems, has been a major goal of early prenatal care since the mid-twentieth century. Since its inception, much—but not all—prenatal testing has focused on uncovering cases of trisomy 21, or Down syndrome, a syndrome in which an embryo, and then a fetus, and then a baby ends up with an extra copy of chromosome number 21. Down syndrome doesn't generally run in families; it can happen to anyone, but its risk increases with maternal age, occurring more frequently when women conceive a pregnancy later in life. Of course, prenatal testing also looks for other genetic conditions, some of which are more serious than Down syndrome and many of which are associated with a baby who can die before or shortly after birth.

When prenatal diagnosis was in its infancy, the capabilities were simple and thus so was the way it was used. In the 1970s, any offer of prenatal testing was reduced to a binary approach: if a pregnant woman was under 35, then often her doctor just didn't discuss the matter, whether she was aged 21 with a 1 in 1,460 risk of Down syndrome or aged 34 with a risk of Down syndrome almost three times as high, at 1 in 456.[1] If she was going to be 35 or older at the time of

delivery, then not only was the possibility of Down syndrome mentioned, but amniocentesis was routinely recommended for its ability
to obtain a complete and precise diagnosis.

Amniocentesis is an invasive procedure wherein a needle is
placed into the uterus to withdraw amniotic fluid for testing; chorionic villus sampling (CVS) is a similar procedure, utilized slightly
earlier in pregnancy, that samples the placenta. Any invasive test,
whether it's amniocentesis or CVS, confers a risk. Any test that
involves putting a needle into the pregnancy to get cells comes with
a chance of losing the pregnancy. That chance is small, somewhere
between 1 in 200 and 1 in 1,000; but it's not zero.[2]

Though it feels extreme now, during that time period, many
women over age 35 were told they "needed" to have an amniocentesis,
that after age 35 it was just shortsighted, maybe even stupid or unsafe,
not to do so. (Even today, many women are still given this message.)

Even back in the 1970s, this age-only screening strategy for prenatal genetic diseases was known to be terribly inadequate. It meant
that more than 5 percent of women would undergo amniocentesis, and yet (because more young women have pregnancies) only
approximately 35 percent of all Down syndrome pregnancies would
be identified.[3]

These days, this reductive duality—amnio or bust—is not how
this discussion is supposed to work. Most guidelines from obstetric
or genetic organizations have long included a recommendation of
screening for multiple genetic conditions to all patients, regardless of
age. That has been possible, in part, because we have an ever-increasing
panel of technologically advanced tools to get us information, each
with its own level of accuracy and its own level of risk.

The revolution started with tests of pregnancy-related chemicals in maternal blood, chemicals made by the placenta. These chemicals often (but not always) go up in the presence of some genetic diseases and often (but not always) go down in others. These chemical markers mean that blood tests from a pregnant woman can be sent to a lab and offer some sort of idea of the risk for Down syndrome and a few other conditions without conferring any risk of miscarriage. The information from these tests was always more of a correlation than a diagnosis. But the possibility of at least some information without risk made them appealing nonetheless.

Shortly thereafter, different chemicals were tested, in different combinations, leading to a proliferation of configurations—triple screen with three chemicals, quad screen with four, penta screen with five—since the 1980s.[4] At the same time, subtle ultrasound signs, also found to be associated with Down syndrome or other genetic diseases, were explored. The most useful of those ultrasound findings has remained the nuchal translucency—the clear space at the back of the fetal neck, measured between 11 and 13+6/7 weeks of pregnancy.

None of these tests have ever been perfect; at their best, they picked up 80 to 90 percent of Down syndrome cases. They also had a false-positive rate of about 5 percent, which meant that a large number of women were flagged as high risk who had absolutely no reason for concern. But despite their inaccuracies, these tests were embraced and recommended because they offered a middle ground; it was a relief not to have only the options of amnio or nothing, and these were a way to avoid increased risk but get a bit of useful information. Because the difficulty understanding what these tests actually can and can't tell us has been clear from the beginning, recommendations for these tests were always accompanied by strongly worded recommendations for genetic counseling and education.

This deeply imperfect science was introduced to the public and has been integral to early pregnancy care ever since. The use of genetic screening has massively increased: we now look for many different genetic conditions, sometimes using our old tests, and every year we have new tests to look for additional diseases.

These genetic diseases are common, and their diagnosis is important. Genetic testing isn't a topic we can avoid. In the right situations, this testing can be incredibly valuable and allow a woman to make choices about her pregnancy and her body that she previously would not have had. But just like that first conversation in the first prenatal visit, it's much easier to leave the complexities behind. Even when I'm able to spend the time and the emotional energy, it's still almost impossible to discuss this topic well.

.   .   .

FOR A LONG time, first-trimester screening (FTS) was the standard of care for genetic diagnosis for patients who didn't want to head straight to an amnio. FTS is a two-part process: it includes a maternal blood test for some of those chemicals made by the placenta, plus an ultrasound to look at the nuchal translucency, completed between 11 and 14 weeks of pregnancy.

Most of the time, an FTS appointment goes something like this: My 2:30 patient, Patricia Seward, is here for a nuchal translucency ultrasound. She doesn't really know why she's here; at her first prenatal visit, the office poked her and took many tubes of blood, and nobody really explained which one was for what. Her doctor mentioned something about genetics screening—maybe he even mentioned Down syndrome—but he mostly seemed to say that the high-risk doctor would take care of this at the ultrasound visit. Patricia doesn't remember why genetics testing is happening at all; there definitely wasn't any conversation about whether or not she wanted any of these tests.

She comes early for her appointment, and her husband is here, too; they both took the time off work because they're excited to see the heartbeat again. The room is chatty, and it's fun to see the fetus moving all over, though the time spent by the technician getting a perfect picture of the back of the fetal neck may seem excessive to Patricia. A bit of stress and some dark tendrils of worry start to creep into the dim ultrasound room.

The measurement of the nuchal translucency is extremely precise; it's hard to do right and very, very easy to do wrong. Today, it's difficult to get the correct picture, so the technician asks Patricia to roll to one side and then the other, but still the angle is wrong, or the fetus is too close to the uterine wall, or there is some other disqualifying detail. The technician ends up coming to get me, and I repeat the maneuvers; I ask Patricia to cough and then be still, but I can't get what we need. I'm about to suggest trying an internal transvaginal ultrasound when the fetus does a quarter flip, and bam, gives me the image I've been fighting for.

I print out our hard-won measurement—1.9 millimeters, normal—and Patricia and her husband and I sit down in my office next door to the ultrasound room. She's done her labs already, and this particular laboratory has an online Web portal, so I log in and input the nuchal translucency measurement and get immediate results on her risk for Down syndrome and two other, more serious, genetic conditions. I print it out and set it in front of the patient and her husband.

Now the hard work starts. I want them to understand what we do and don't know; what we can and can't say. I know her doctor didn't do any of this, so I try to explain: "The nuchal translucency was normal. The blood test was normal. Your test gives a risk of Down syndrome of 1 in 922; it gives you a risk of trisomy 13 or 18 of 1 in over 10,000." The numbers generated by this test are always ridiculously, misleadingly precise, granting an illusion of certainty that is extremely hard to overcome.

I show Patricia and her husband the paper with her results; I show them the bar graph demonstrating that her risk is lower than that predicted by her age—equivalent now to that of a 20-year-old!—but that it's not zero. I review that the test is imperfect and that even reassuring results are not the whole story. At this point, Patricia and her husband are quiet. Her husband clears his throat: "I'm sorry, doctor. Are you telling us good news or bad news?"

They're confused; I clearly haven't been doing as good a job as I thought. I try to make it clear; I smile; I soften my voice. "This is usually good news," I say. "Most people stop here. It's just not certain news, so I want you to know that if you wanted to know more securely, we could get more information. We could do more tests, including invasive ones with a needle." The mention of the needle is recognized and almost immediately provokes some frantic hand-waving. No, no, no, no needles, thank you very much, we're so happy, see you in a few months at the 18-week anatomy scan.

Patricia and her husband walk out with their paperwork that has complicated, uncertain numbers on it, and they say to each other, "Everything's fine."

In the end, my counseling session is reduced to those two words: "Everything's fine." And they're almost entirely right: everything is, probably, fine. If expectant parents aren't going to do anything to make that "probably" into a "definitely," then why not just delete it from the sentence and let them enjoy the pregnancy?

. . .

FOR MOST PEOPLE, the fact that everything is probably fine will eventually translate into everything *is* fine—because the vast majority of babies are born healthy in this amazing human system of ours. But somewhere, someone is affected by a terrible diagnosis, even if she, too, thought it happened only to other people. The odds for her and for her fetus become one in every one, and that one is here, today, now. On that day, there may or may not be a choice to make or an action to take.

Deleting that "probably" from my counseling session gives the illusion that there are no actions that can be taken, no choices that can be made; the patient is allowed to decline all my counseling if she wants. But what seems more common and is much worse is when the doctor declines to do the counseling: we delete any discussion of what testing we've done or haven't done; we don't discuss what we're looking for or what tests we've elected to omit. Leaving that vacuum within prenatal counseling takes any power from the patient and gives it to the doctor. By default, it checks all the "no" boxes for her without asking her. But nobody except this woman and her chosen decision team can know what the answers would be. And even she can only know that answer with more information.

Here's some of that information: 3 to 6 percent of all newborns have an abnormality. Some of those are small—a cleft palate, a small heart defect, a club foot. But others are much, much bigger: an extra chromosome here, a lost gene there. Some of them, though, defy imagination. Did you know that the brain might not form, leaving a fluid-filled globe of skull? Or that the heart can grow outside the body? Or that some bones might be made of a delicate glass-like substance, breaking dozens of times before the fetus is even born?

It turns out that there are more things in heaven and earth than are dreamt of in your philosophy, but also more in your own pregnancy, in your own body.

Sometimes these diagnoses—like a cleft palate—can be easily remedied in early life. Other diagnoses will mean a difficult life but perhaps an enjoyable one. Others mean a life full of pain. Even others mean a short life, sometimes death before birth or within the first few days of life. Some families find that they can tolerate one reality but not another; others have to guess at what their family would be like, what their life would be like; what their joy would be like and their burden; their other children's lives, their finances, their marriage, their work, their community. The calculus is complex, and the variables change with every test, every ultrasound, every expert consulted.

Thus, it's almost impossible to know what any family might choose. Many women start the process by saying they'd never have an abortion, no matter what, no way. But some of those families learn a new vocabulary, one that exceeds the limits they had previously understood to be possible. There is more than is dreamt of in your philosophy: there is heaven and earth; but we need to mention that there's hell, too.

It's so much easier not to talk about these possibilities. It's so easy to leave it as "everything is fine"; because everything probably is fine. But if everything isn't fine, then the patient never had a moment to understand what was going on; by withholding the possibility of unpleasant information, the provider also withholds the choice.

Not only is the decision to terminate a pregnancy in these situations difficult and nearly always drenched in sorrow; it also has an expiration date. In most of the United States, termination of pregnancy can only be offered until fetal viability—somewhere close to 24 weeks (see Chapter 5). Earlier procedures, those prior to 14 weeks, are safer for the mom and easier to endure—1-day procedures rather than 2- or 3-day ordeals of cervical dilation and operating room time. Time is the enemy; as the days and weeks tick by, options are lost, procedural risk goes up, heartbreaks mount.

. . .

AURA VALDEZ ALREADY knew; she told me the day I met her. She has one child with a disability—something about his brain didn't develop properly. It's an unusual diagnosis; at some point in development, his brain surface just never folded. On his prenatal ultrasounds, six years ago, the brain never developed into the cauliflower shape that we normally see; it stayed smooth, like an egg, she told me. She knew during the pregnancy that something wasn't right; our doctors had told her that the brain didn't look normal. She didn't agree to an amnio in that pregnancy or consider termination. She didn't really know what this brain smoothness would mean then; she hoped for the best and carried on.

But she can tell me what it means now: her child is almost 5 but has never smiled; he's never rolled over or crawled. She is told that he will never talk. He has the most beautiful hazel eyes, and in the picture she carries with her, he is in a lovely new Christmas sweater. She spends her days with him, which means she can't work; most of her time is spent caring for him or filling out forms and making phone calls to get care for him. Her husband works a lot, since she can't, so she's almost always alone with her son. Finding a sitter who can manage her son's medical needs so she can do anything for herself is a challenge. But she managed today, because today is important.

Aura is pregnant again, around 16 weeks. It was unplanned, which meant we didn't have a chance to discuss any prepregnancy ways to avoid potential problems. (This is probably moot, because almost all of the available methods would involve in vitro fertilization so that we could diagnose the embryo before implantation; this would be beyond the coverage of her insurance and well beyond her financial means.) But she knew she had to come early for her anatomy scan, and yesterday she had the first look at the brain. It wasn't definitive, but the brain already didn't look quite normal. Because this time we know what we're looking for—since we have a diagnosis from her 5-year-old—at the time of ultrasound we have a very specific test via amnio available, a way to look for the particular genetic error that her 5-year-old has. This time, Aura didn't wait for us to offer; she came in asking for invasive testing. Now she's here at the ultrasound suite, after a lot of counseling, but mostly she's just sad: "I already know, I think. And we can't do this again."

I counsel her about the risks and benefits of her amniocentesis, and we sign all the forms together. I confirm her name, her date of birth, her blood type—she's B positive, and the genetic counselor makes a dumb joke: "That's my favorite blood type, you know? Because we have to be positive?" Aura smiles tightly, and nobody laughs.

Then I turn off all the lights; we are in a dim twilight, lit only by the ultrasound machine's bright fuzz, starry skies on a television screen. Aura lies back on the narrow bed, slightly tilted upward. The very experienced ultrasound technician scans the belly, and together we find a likely spot for the needle; no placenta, no fetus, just empty black space. I quickly mark the skin with my ballpoint pen.

Aura doesn't have anyone with her today, so the medical student observing me sits in the chair by the side of the bed and offers to hold her hand if it would be helpful. Aura doesn't say anything but takes the student's right hand and holds it tight. I ask her to put her other hand behind her head, both to keep it out of the way and to relax the abdominal muscles.

I put on my sterile gloves. I swab the belly with the scratchy sponges soaked in brown disinfectant—once, twice, three times. I place sterile drapes, one on top, one on the bottom, one on each side. They cover all of Aura's belly except a small rectangle, at the center of which is the tiny dot from my ballpoint pen, an altar facing the sky, all that she can sacrifice, exposed.

The tech puts the ultrasound probe under the drapes, angled so that he can show me where I am. While watching closely on the ultrasound machine, I insert my needle, right in the middle of the small, barely convex rectangle of belly left uncovered. The tech shows me where my needle is, shining brightly on the ultrasound screen, sparkling in the image as it scatters the sound waves, moving forward through a layer of maternal fat, through the muscle, and into the uterine wall.

We confirm that we are still in a good spot—far from fetus, far from placenta—and with a final pop, I push through the uterine wall into the amniotic sac. I withdraw the hard needle guide from within the needle and quickly attach a small syringe. I withdraw 2 milliliters of yellow fluid for us to discard as possibly contaminated with maternal blood, and then, without shaking, I attach a new syringe and withdraw 25 milliliters of clear yellow amniotic fluid, which will be sent for diagnosis. I unscrew the syringe and lay it on my instrument table and then remove the needle from the belly. We're done.

I hold down a sterile gauze at the site of the needle insertion. With my other hand, I show the patient the vial of amniotic fluid: yellow, no blood: a clean tap. The tech shows her the fetus, moving around, unaware of our visit. "Looks like we didn't bother anyone!" We check the fetal heart rate quickly: boom–boom boom–boom, 140 beats per minute, normal. The whole procedure lasted less than 2 minutes.

I put a bandage on the site of the amniocentesis; it always surprises people that the wound is so small for a procedure over which we agonize so much. The patient sits up, and I walk her to our small recovery area. I review that she should call us for severe cramping or fever or leaking of fluid from the vagina; I review the recommendations for the rest of the day—no heavy lifting, no sex. I wonder if she has to lift her 5-year-old later today, but she doesn't ask me about it. She sits in the brown recliner in the windowless recovery room and closes her eyes. When I come back after the next patient, she's already left.

Aura's results come back a week later, positive for the same genetic error that her son has. She meets with our genetic counselors and opts for termination, as soon as possible, please. She finds care for her son and comes in on a Friday for her procedure. My colleague from family planning tells me later that Aura had an uncomplicated pregnancy termination. She asked for a memento from the fetus, as many women do; in the operating room, the team was able to make tiny footprints for her to have, to keep after the termination. The doctor offered her, and Aura gratefully accepted, an IUD placement at the time of termination. "Five years sounded about right to her," my colleague said. "I told her we can always remove it earlier. But she said she has to wait a good long while before she wants to even think about trying again."

I ask my office to reach out to Aura; they give her an appointment for pre-conception counseling so that we can discuss how to avoid this situation in a future pregnancy. Aura doesn't keep her appointment and declines to reschedule when our office staff calls her again.

. . .

TERMINATION IS ONE way to handle a terrible diagnosis, but it's not the only way. For those patients who don't want to terminate, who want to continue a pregnancy with a diagnosed problem, the ability to get a precise diagnosis is arguably even more important. Without information, deliveries happen without preparation, leading to very sick babies born in hospitals without the capability to give them the care they need: babies that turn blue after delivery, with no doctor ready to resuscitate.

If we know what challenges a newborn will face—and if the family has had time to better decide what they want—we can make sure the delivery happens at a hospital that has the right surgical team available; we can make sure that, right at delivery, the baby has a team to help it breathe without delay. We can take the time during the pregnancy to introduce the family to the cardiologist and the neurologist and the renal specialist; this family can have a team and a plan and start working together, even before the birth.

And in some of the most truly awful situations, we can discuss how to limit the awfulness. Should we do a cesarean delivery for a persistently breech baby or for a baby who is not tolerating labor if the baby will die soon after labor? Can we keep the room quiet and less chaotic and give a family the time they can have with their baby, even if it won't be very long? For one family, knowing that their baby would die from underdeveloped lungs soon after birth meant that we made sure the patient had adequate pain management very early in her labor. We disconnected all the fetal monitors and made sure to leave them alone with their baby after birth. They had 2 hours together before the baby died. Years later, the patient has said that those 2 hours remain unimaginably precious to her, a source of tremendous comfort.

Those 2 hours were granted to her by the flawed and powerful tools of prenatal diagnosis. The information that our tools obtained was catastrophic, but the knowledge of it beforehand allowed this family to claim the only time they would have together, to know that it was their only time while it was happening. Without that information, those 2 hours would have been a frenzy of panic, doctors, needles, pain, more doctors. That time would almost have definitely been spent apart. Those 2 hours were a terrible, beautiful, irreplaceable gift.

Prenatal diagnosis isn't only for people who would terminate pregnancy. It is, however, useful only for patients who are ready to know that Bad Things are out there, who are ready to discuss that the boogeyman is real. It's hard enough to have a discussion about prenatal diagnosis when the results are normal; it's hard enough to understand an FTS when it's not alarming. But when the results aren't normal, that's even harder to listen to. And in those situations, the mismatch between what a patient is willing to know and what the doctor can tell them can lead to real trouble.

What can be done when patients don't want to know everything they can? What do we do when people don't want to think about the Bad Things that might be lurking within their own body?

. . .

DeeAnn was young and pregnant and came to her first-trimester ultrasound to get a cute picture of the baby. I had never met her before. DeeAnn brought her best friend and her boyfriend, and the room was boisterous with yells and laughter, so loud that I could hear them down the hall.

When the tech put the ultrasound probe on, she spent only a minute or two getting pictures. She was supposed to get that picture of the back of the fetal neck, the nuchal translucency. But the tech only scanned for a moment because she didn't even need to measure to know that something was very wrong. The back of the fetal neck was swollen; actually, so was the whole back of the fetal body, with striations crisscrossing the fluid-filled area. This kind of abnormality is called a septated cystic hygroma and is very frequently found with several genetic syndromes; but even if genetics are normal, there's a strong association with cardiac and other problems. With just this one look, our ultrasound showed that this patient had an 83 percent chance of having either a pregnancy loss or a very abnormal baby.[5]

The tech came to fetch me, and we walked back to the room together. Already, DeeAnn could see that something wasn't quite right; the room got very quiet. I scanned her belly for several minutes, trying to gather more clues. Then I asked DeeAnn to sit up and talk to me. I asked her if she wanted privacy. She said no; she wanted her friends to stay.

I began with my usual sentence to start the discussion of a fetal anomaly: "I am concerned about something I see on the ultrasound." In that room, I was met with complete silence. I took a deep breath and started to explain about the back of the neck, about what it could mean, about testing for genetic issues. But I didn't get far before DeeAnn interrupted me. She leaned forward. "My baby's perfect," she said to me.

"I hope that's true. But I do see something here that isn't quite normal, and I'd like to at least discuss what it might mean."

"My baby is *perfect*. My baby has nothing wrong. Nothing. You doctors always just want to do more tests."

Back and forth we went for a little while; she didn't want to talk about going to counseling or about further testing options or even what the diagnoses might be. I didn't even get to mention amniocentesis or CVS. Every time I started to say something about the ultrasound, DeeAnn cut me off. She told me I was trying to make money off of her and her pregnancy; that I wanted tests so that I could get paid for them. The only sentence she wanted to hear from me was that everything was fine. But that was the one thing I couldn't truthfully say.

The conversation didn't last long. DeeAnn's voice rose, and I'm sure mine did, too. DeeAnn told me she was leaving and that she would report me to the hospital as a "bad doctor" on her way out. She demanded a picture from the ultrasound "to put on my fridge," and I printed out the picture we had—barely recognizable as a fetus, clearly abnormal to educated eyes. She grabbed it from my hand and left with her friends behind her.

It was, frankly, a terrible appointment. I felt like a failure: I couldn't get beyond her rejection. I also knew—or I thought I knew—that she would regret our abbreviated conversation. DeeAnn so quickly jettisoned me and any knowledge I could give her; she didn't wait to learn that some of the answers we could get for her might shape the management of her pregnancy.

But she didn't want any of that information. Her general approach to our appointment seemed based on mistrust of me mixed with hopeful delusion. When that potent mixture crashed against what I was trying to tell her, it became a huge wave of anger. I couldn't get beyond the anger, and I thought that the main victim of that anger was the patient herself.

Later, I was less sure that she was wrong. To some extent, prenatal diagnosis is about the conflict between the generalities that diagnoses require—the technical labels that are required to discuss things like "profound intellectual disability" or "inconsistent with a normal life span"—and the profound particularism of parental love: "This is my one child, one in the whole world; I wouldn't change a hair on her head and I'll hurt anyone who dares try."

That's the work that happens as we become parents. We chemically alter the general to the particular, until one day we are left with our baby, our child, our one and only. For some of us, that day is when we see two lines on a pregnancy test stick; for others, it's when we feel the fetus move; for still others, it's at delivery. And for some of us, it is weeks or months after delivery. But for DeeAnn, perhaps that work was done much much earlier.

From that perspective, DeeAnn's approach made some sense. She had come to our ultrasound suite for a fetal photo session. She wasn't interested in a medical diagnostic scan; she was interested in getting mementos from a pregnancy that she was already deeply invested in. She hadn't come to me for a diagnosis; she had come to me for celebration.

I've always been on the side of finding out more information. That's what doctors do—and scientists and academics and avid readers. I am all those people; I seek out information, usually with irresistible force. During that meeting with DeeAnn, she clearly identified information as a liability in this situation; she rejected it all. What happened in that ultrasound room is what always happens when an irresistible force meets an immovable object: collision.

It took my own traumatic experience to learn that maybe Dee-Ann was a tiny bit right, to become my own immovable object. Sometimes, as DeeAnn already knew, more information doesn't enrich us; it can beggar us. I had to learn this myself, the hard way.

About a decade ago, a new tool in prenatal diagnosis was developed, different from anything that had come before, called cell-free DNA testing or noninvasive prenatal testing (NIPT). It goes by a large number of brand names—Harmony, Panorama, Maternity21—all selling essentially the same thing, and it may, one day, change everything.

NIPT is a test that provides fetal DNA—the same DNA we were looking for in cells procured from amniocentesis and CVS—but gets it from maternal blood. NIPT looks at the DNA floating freely in maternal blood that's not in cells. Most of that DNA is maternal, but a small percentage is fetal, from the placental cells that are in contact with the maternal blood supply.[6]

The DNA that NIPT can look at from the placental cells is never a full chromosome; it's always just bits and pieces. But NIPT means that the lab can take those bits and pieces, isolate them, multiply them, and do math with them. It's a bit like taking the residue from your garbage disposal and figuring out whether there were two or three people over for dinner and how many of them had mashed potatoes. NIPT can look and ask, "Are there too many bits of chromosome 21?"

NIPT is still being studied; right now, we have data showing that it can identify around 98 to 99 percent of all Down syndrome pregnancies in high-risk populations.[7] In low-risk pregnancies, it's not yet clear if it's actually better than the first-trimester screening we were already using. One day, though, it might have the potential to be even better and smarter—to give us some of the certainty we've always been searching for without having to trade it for the risks of invasive testing. But we're not there right now.

.   .   .

WHEN I WAS 38, I became pregnant. We had wanted another child for a long time, and my joke was that it was my chance at a geriatric pregnancy, but it was a joke made in gratitude and relief—I was just so happy to be pregnant. But because I was so very advanced in maternal age, I followed my own advice and went to seek out NIPT testing. If I could've, I would have had it drawn at my own office, but at the time NIPT was a new and restricted test, only available through our genetic counselors.

While I was at the genetic counselors, they noted that my Ashkenazi Jewish testing was outdated.

"But I just got it done three years ago," I protested.

"Nonetheless," they said, "We expanded it from 19 to 38 possible diseases. You should really get them all tested."

"Sure," I said. "I'm always negative. Good stock. I always tell my husband how lucky he was to marry me."

Two weeks later, my NIPT results came back with low risk for Down syndrome. I had completely forgotten that we had also sent out the expanded Ashkenazi Jewish panel. I was 14 weeks pregnant, and I thought I had all the information I needed to take a deep breath. With the normal NIPT in hand, we told our older kids that a baby was on the way. We explained why Mama was so tired and sick but still so very happy.

Three days later, the genetic counselor called me:

"Your results are abnormal."

"No." I said. "No, I saw. My NIPT was normal—I got it back already."

"Um, no, not the NIPT. Your Ashkenazi Jewish panel. You're a carrier for a genetic disease."

Of the 38 diseases, the one I tested positive for—let's call it problem X—was one that, if also carried by my husband, gave us a 25 percent chance of having an affected baby. If we both had problem X on our genes and both gave it to this pregnancy, then we would have a baby that would likely die before the age of 3 and whose short life would be marked by pain and suffering.

As I got off the phone with the genetic counselor, I didn't know what to say or what to feel. I can't even tell you if I knew at that point whether I would have considered termination of pregnancy for a baby that would have such a short, painful life. Stupid, stupid me had thought we were beyond these issues, so I didn't have any thoughts at all.

The next step would be to test my husband. He came in with me the next day to have his blood drawn. And then we waited. We waited 1 week, then 2, then 3 agonizing weeks.

During those 3 weeks, I remained shut down. I couldn't talk, and I couldn't really think. I was still nauseated all the time; I was still tired all the time; but now I was also terrified. For those weeks, I clenched my jaw and opened my eyes and went through my days.

I went to work and came home; bathed my kids and emptied the dishwasher. I ate, and I threw up, and I waited for the days to pass. When my 5-year-old asked about the pregnancy inside my belly, something about my face must have shut him down, too; I didn't even have enough words left to reassure him. It only took once or twice before he stopped asking.

My husband's results finally came back. He was "likely negative" for problem X but—surprise!—positive for problem Y. And, it turned out, upon review, neither of the tests that we had undergone for either problem X or problem Y were completely perfect—both had about a 5 percent chance of being falsely reassuring. In other words, there was about a 1 in 20 chance that he did carry problem X or that I did carry problem Y. And any problem that we both had could give us a fatally ill baby.

The genetic counselors offered us a second test for problem X, a plan to sequence the gene for each base pair. Oh, we could also do it for problem Y if we wanted to! It was recently developed! It would cost $3,000 and take about a month, but would be pretty close to definitive. Unless perhaps we'd like to consider an amniocentesis? We could do that, too, and directly check the fetal cells; that would cost $3,000 and take a month, too.

At some point during this conversation, I looked at my husband and said, "I don't think I can survive another month like this one. I think we're done here." As the counselor talked more and more about the numbers—smaller and smaller but never zero—of terrible things happening, I told my husband I wanted to stop.

What I really meant was this: We're far enough from disease that I think we get to choose. I am choosing. I choose to be reassured. I choose to ignore the fact that I can have more information;

I choose to go home and celebrate the information we do have with our family. I choose to go home and reclaim my joy. I am choosing to have this baby.

And I did. And she is wonderful.

But I remember, now, the foolishness I felt for having gotten tests that I didn't want; for having information that, in lieu of helping me, stole from me the joy in my pregnancy, in my healthy children; that cut me in half for a month.

This information—even the possibility of this information—damaged us deeply, despite the fact that I knew what I was getting into and that I understood the numbers. This liability—information that harms without helping—is what DeeAnn rejected. Is that liability a large part of what I'm offering my patients at that first prenatal visit?

Here's what we've known since we started telling the story of how Eve bit the apple: knowledge is powerful and painful and damaging, but it's also powerful and healing and wonderful. Because knowledge can cut both ways, it is better that any human should wield it for herself, better that it not be wielded by anyone else for her. And ignorance is powerful too; it's a vacuum that gets filled by someone else's decisions.

If I could do it all over again, would I reject the Ashkenazi Jewish testing? Ultimately, that test was meaningless; my daughter is fine and would have been if I had not undergone any prenatal diagnosis at all. But if I could do it all over again, I wouldn't reject that knowledge. I would do the Ashkenazi testing, but earlier, before the pregnancy, before I had a very firm reality growing in my body. I would rather know; I just would want to choose the conditions of my knowing. And of course, if the outcome were different, if the pregnancy wasn't healthy, then I would want to know that, too. Because choosing ignorance also creates decisions and makes a reality: it just means that someone else would be making them for me.

Even if nothing changes, the knowledge is powerful. Even if the world keeps on turning in exactly the same way, knowing how you fit in the story can sometimes be the beginning of healing.

. . .

I WAS COMING into work for the night shift, and my partner asked me to check on a patient in the postanesthesia recovery room—to sign her discharge papers and send her home if she was doing okay postoperatively.

The patient had been followed by the GYN team for a while; she had come in for a little bit of spotting at 11 weeks gestation, and even on our terrible little emergency room ultrasound, multiple abnormalities had been noted. Her fetus had empty space where the front of the brain should have been; there was also a strange protuberance in the forehead area called a proboscis. The fetus was also very small for gestational age and had not been growing well.

Together, these features suggested trisomy 13, a syndrome with three copies of chromosome 13 that is associated with abnormalities throughout the body and an extremely poor prognosis. Many of these pregnancies end in miscarriage; of those that live to deliver, fewer than 20 percent live past the first few days or weeks of life. The diagnosis on the National Institutes of Health (NIH) descriptive page for trisomy 13 uses the phrase "severe intellectual disability" several times.[8]

The patient's bleeding had stopped, but she desperately wanted to know what was going on. Her doctors offered her a CVS; she knew that CVS had a very slim chance of causing her to lose the preg-

nancy; she also knew that she was extremely likely to lose the pregnancy in any case. She strongly wanted the CVS.

The results came back and confirmed the guess a week later: trisomy 13. Five days later, almost 2 weeks after the CVS, the patient
came into the emergency department bleeding heavily. She had lost
most of the pregnancy at home, but her bleeding was heavy enough
that she ended up needing to go to the operating room for a dilation
and curettage (D&C) procedure to finish cleaning out her uterus
and stop the bleeding. My partner had finished her surgery shortly
before I found him for signout.

The D&C was uncomplicated, my partner said. The patient had
bled before the procedure but had been very stable since then. If her
vitals were okay and she felt good, she could be discharged home.

A few hours later, I went to the recovery room of the day surgery
unit, almost deserted by 7 p.m. I waved to the nurse at the nursing
station and then started walking down the dim aisle, past curtained,
empty gurneys. Echoing in the darkness, I heard a woman's voice,
calmly talking: "Mama, you know. They say it was a one in ten thousand chance. You know, like winning the lottery, but in a bad way.
They say it's just bad luck; it shouldn't happen again next time. The
doctor said we can try again in a few months."

The patient was fluent in the facts of her particular tragedy. She
had information, and with it, she was talking her way through tragedy into grief; into a sadness that didn't manifest itself in bitterness,
but rather one that can be handled, can be turned over and around,
that can be visited and viewed; a sadness without the poisonous bite
of anger or blame.

On the one hand, the diagnosis of trisomy 13 had changed
nothing. The patient had been losing a pregnancy; once she had a

diagnosis, she continued to lose the pregnancy. But listening to her talk on the phone, I could hear that the diagnosis of trisomy 13 had changed everything. The diagnosis allowed this woman access to a narrative. It also gave her access to our knowledge of thousands of other patients who had been through similar stories: it gave her context and company. It gave also gave her the comfort of knowing that there can be a different ending and that she would likely find her way there.

I stopped at her bed. The patient had red eyes; it looked like she had cried, but she wasn't crying now. "How are you doing?" I asked. I felt her belly, I checked the pad she was wearing; I eyeballed her vital signs.

"I had something bad happen. But I'm going to be okay. Can I go home?"

"Yeah. Let's get you out of here. You're going to be fine."

SECOND TRIMESTER

4.

Anatomy Ultrasound

Incidentalomas

Her Facebook status says: "Is it too much to ask for our medical providers to treat us like human beings?" Five people have already left a little sad face and three more have "liked" the post. The rest of her comment discusses what happened: a doctor who didn't ask her name made a slightly off-color joke and ended by using some derogatory words to discuss her weight.

Her Facebook comments fill up quickly: other women saying yep, that happened to me, or much worse. Other comments come from physician friends who try to point out that the medical system is dysfunctional, with short visit times, overburdened providers, and emotional burnout, leading to this kind of apathetic behavior. Predictably, none of those comments are received well.

I start writing a comment. It would be wiser to be quiet than comment—isn't it always?—but she's talking about my work, my world, and she's my friend. I start a comment offering to refer her to a great OBGYN I know in her neighborhood. I backspace the whole thing and start to write about how the doctor was kind of a jerk, but that thankfully no actual malpractice was committed, so I guess it could be worse; I delete that before I even get to the end. I begin a sentence about how almost all professional groups recommend that we discuss weight and obesity at all visits,[1] so that avoiding the discussion is kind of being a bad doctor, but entering that discussion in a positive, shame-free way is almost impossible. I delete that.

What I can't write is that I've been both the patient of a doctor who said those things and the doctor who said those things; I've been the victim and the perpetrator. What I can't write is that talking to people—really talking to people—is so hard to do well and so easy to do wrong. Doctors and patients think we're both speaking the same language, but we're not, we haven't been for years.

Finally, I write this: "I'm so sorry. We all deserve better and I hope you get it." It's inadequate, but at least it's not a lie.

.   .   .

IF YOU ASKED me what language I speak at work, I would say that I'm speaking English. Technically, that's true, but if I were to be precise, what I'm really speaking is Medical Language, the official language of Doctor. All of us in Doctor read and write Regular Person English; after all, we grew up in Regular Person and still live there most of the time.

Somehow, during the process that turns us into doctors, we start speaking differently. We start talking in Medical Language; we become fluent in it. The first two years of medical school are largely consumed by trying to internalize textbooks' worth of Medical Language. In the first days of medical school, doctors-to-be learn words for the body's anatomy: words for muscles and bones and vessels and nerves that we never knew and words for the way they branch and connect.

Sometimes the Medical Language words we learn aren't even words; many of them are silly or often filthy acronyms, invented to remember sheer masses of information—the branches of arteries off the aorta or the kinds of nerves that innervate the penis. Like any language, Medical Language is dynamic: it has slang, it has jokes, it has neologisms. One of my favorites is "incidentaloma," a mash-up of an incidental finding—something you find that you're not looking for—and the ending "oma," which means a swelling or a tumor. So if the CT scan that was ordered to look for a lung clot finds a small fibrous mass near the diaphragm, that's an incidentaloma. (But now the race for figuring it out has begun. Is it old tuberculosis? Prior trauma? New cancer?) Nobody would ever use this word in a formal radiology report—it's casual and somewhat dismissive—but it helpfully connotes the frustration of finding something unrelated to the problem you need to solve, but one that is going to cause the patient (and to a much smaller extent, the doctor) a lot of stress and follow-up testing anyway.

Medical Language includes a different way of thinking; medical students learn ways to interpret and translate what patients are telling them. Medical Language is designed to surgically extract what a doctor needs to know from what they've been told. When the patient says she feels light-headed, does she mean she feels vertiginous, that she feels the room is actually spinning, likely a neurological or inner ear problem? Or does she mean she feels like she's about to faint—presyncope? The latter is more concerning for a feeling that accompanies an abrupt fall in blood pressure.

Knowing which one the patient means is not just a linguistic distinction: it's a concrete difference in the reality of what she's describing and determines whether to worry about a seizure or about dehydration. In that surgical extraction of meaning by Medical Language, there is the introduction of something new: a distance between the patient and her own perceptions, her own feelings, her own body. Medical Language takes "patient writhing in labor and begging for epidural" and makes it into "patient reports moderate distress, requesting analgesia."

That's only the first part of how Medical Language takes information that a patient provides and subjects it to interpretation. There is a whole subset of Medical Language that describes how to think and how to organize information. Medical students learn to "take a history and a physical" when we meet a patient, a shorthand way of referring to all the information gathered within an appointment. Much of the entire third year of medical school is learning how to appropriately write SOAP notes. SOAP stands for Subjective (what the patient says), Objective (what the doctor observes, including the physical exam, lab results, and radiology results), which leads to the Assessment (what the doctor thinks is going on), and Plan (what the doctor and patient want to do about it). SOAP notes are as strict a format as some forms of Elizabethan poetry; what is excluded can be as important as what is included. The end result, the SOAP notes, is a tight, efficient piece of prose, a transfer of enormous amounts of complex information, often in less than a page.

After all, this is the first purpose of Medical Language, the stated purpose. It allows those of us occupied in assessing and caring for the human body the language to properly do so. It reduces the complexity of the human body and experience to hard, classifiable details.

This language allows us the technical, concrete expression necessary to explain to each other exactly where and how to put a scalpel through human skin; why the expensive and risky medication was necessary; why the patient needs to be transferred to the ICU immediately.

Medical Language allows communication not just today, in the present, with our colleagues. The language can go across space and time and access all the experiences that came before us. That is, the right Medical Language accesses knowledge. And without it, we can be lost.

. . .

ONE WEDNESDAY MORNING, I am in one of the ultrasound offices, entering a room to review an anatomy scan. For these appointments, though I've read through the patient's chart previously, this entrance into the dark ultrasound room is usually how I end up meeting the patient herself. This patient, Eleanor Kovac, has already spent about 30 minutes with the technician, who has taken over 100 pictures in order to get us the 80 that we need; the tech then excuses herself to get me.

When I come into the room, it's still dark; the tech has kept the lights off. I come in quietly and head to the sink to wash my hands. Eleanor is lying on the table; her husband is sitting in the chair to her left so they can both see the oversized TV screen in the far corner where everything I see on my screen shows up for them, too. I introduce myself and ask a few questions about Eleanor's health, her pregnancy, what she knows so far. Eleanor seems businesslike but also new to this: it's her first baby. She's here straight from her workplace, with sensible heels kicked off to the side of the bed and a trim blouse hiked up over her belly so that it won't get stained by the gel we use to scan.

The ultrasound Eleanor is here for today is called "the anatomy scan"; it's the big 18-to-20-week scan that helps us know if there are any major malformations in the fetus. I often refer to it as the fetus's first doctor visit, and it's one of the most complex studies we do.

After I talk with Eleanor, I start scrolling through the pictures the tech took; as usual, they're beautiful work. Together, the pictures tell me an anatomic story of a healthy fetus. I try to narrate what I'm seeing as I flip through the pictures, but I also tell Eleanor and her husband that the concentration required for this kind of visual work allows me little room for speech, so I tend to trail off a bit. Everything does look good, but there are a few parts of the fetal abdomen the tech asked me to try to get; she wasn't able to get a clear picture because of the way the fetal spine was blocking.

When I'm done scrolling through the pictures, I pick up the ultrasound probe and take a quick look through the fetus, just to make sure. As I do, I scroll through the brain, the spine, the abdomen . . . wait a second. I see something in the fetal stomach. What is that? Is it just a weird angle? Nope, I scan back and forth, and it's really there, on all my angles. It's . . . debris. Schmutz. A mass? In the fetal stomach? Despite all my years of training and performing fetal ultrasound, I don't think I've ever seen this before.

I can hear that I'm not talking anymore, that I've trailed off and off into a longer silence. I know this is scary so I try to murmur something, tell them I just need a second, a moment to look around.

I'm thinking hard and fast: a mass in the stomach. What is it? Right now, I need to figure out if this stomach mass is a problem: will it hurt a neonate or require surgery? And even if what I'm seeing is not something that will damage the stomach's ability to function, sometimes it's important anyway, a clue to a bigger problem. Prenatal ultrasound is like that: a mystery that sometimes provides only one clue, or sometimes none at all, to a health problem that would be obvious after birth. So, maybe this is some variant of duodenal atresia, which would alert me to a higher chance of Down syndrome in this pregnancy? Or maybe it's some weird gastric bleed and associated with other bleeding issues for this fetus? Or a tumor? I've seen other tumors prenatally—adrenal, cardiac— but I've never heard of a prenatal gastric tumor, so is that even something that occurs? Or maybe this mass is not itself abnormal but a functional issue: some backup, a sign of slow gastric emptying, and therefore a sign of something that would affect intestinal movement, like cystic fibrosis?

Eleanor's husband asks, "Doctor, is there a problem?" I look over, and I see that Eleanor is clutching his hand. I need to know what to tell them, and I don't want to lie. I look around the fetus again: fingers, toes, heart, brain, intestines, placenta. All look really . . . normal. The fetus is growing well. I run through the patient's prenatal genetic testing in my mind: all reassuring, though she didn't do an amniocentesis or CVS, so nothing definitive.

I clear my throat; I say: "Almost everything looks perfect, but there's one thing I want to check out." I know what I've said is not terribly comforting. I am trying to keep my voice relaxed because I don't really know if we have a problem yet. I can hear in the silence Eleanor's unasked questions. I turn to face them more completely; I say, "Why don't you get dressed and come down the hall? We'll chat once you're ready."

I step out of the room and make a dash to the nearest computer to e-mail the head of ultrasound. While typing, I call my partner, who's at the main academic hospital. "Oh, yeah," she says. "It's something I've seen. It's rare, but it's not important. Don't worry about it."

"Ok. Weird that I've never come across it then. What is it called?"

"Dunno. Don't remember. But I have asked about it, and it's no big deal. I'll find you a reference later. Don't worry about it."

When I get off the phone with her, there's already an e-mail back from my ultrasound chair. "Not clinically concerning," he writes. "Don't worry about it."

"But what *is* it?" I type back.

He doesn't respond right away.

I trust my colleagues, but without a name for this thing, "Don't worry about it" isn't advice I can follow. Without language, I'm not able to let it go; I'm also not able to talk about it with the patient. I want terminology; I want a search term, a file label, a hashtag.

I swivel around at the computer and take a few minutes to hunt around journal articles and textbooks. I quickly find several publications describing my finding as a "gastric pseudo-mass."[2] The pictures in the articles look exactly like my pictures. The articles explain that in the second and third trimesters, debris can be visualized in the fetal stomach and is probably swallowed cells (either red blood cells or meconium, fetal bowel contents) that have aggregated due to the usual slow gastric emptying noted in this time period during pregnancy.

Each article I find ends with some version of this: "Gastric pseudo-masses resolve over time and are not associated with adverse neonatal outcome. Therefore, further evaluation of the gastric pseudo-mass is not required."

In other words, "Don't worry about it."

Now that I have language for this finding, I can finally follow that advice. With that terminology, I now know that other doctors have seen this, other ultrasounds have found this, and I can assess whether their knowledge is now applicable to my patient. I can look into the future and see how those babies did once they were born, and I can know that this gastric pseudo-mass did not affect those lives, didn't portend any other serious conditions, didn't mean I had missed anything else important. I have Medical Language for what I saw, and because of that, I can see into the past and into the future.

I meet the patient and her husband in my office, less than 10 minutes since I left them in the ultrasound room. Eleanor is dressed in her office clothes, but her blouse is untucked, her hair still mussed from lying down; she didn't take the few seconds to stop at the mirror. She is sitting in the chair across from my desk, twisting the long ribbon of pictures from the ultrasound in her hands into a winding thread. Her husband is still standing, shifting his weight from foot to foot.

I sit down, and Eleanor's husband does as well. I smile and say, "Everything is really okay. I'm sorry I worried you." I pull up one of the articles on gastric pseudo-mass on my computer screen. I show Eleanor and her husband the picture of the stomach from their scan, and I show them the picture from the articles; I tell her what we saw and how it's not clinically significant. I tell them that there are no guarantees in fetal ultrasound, but that absolutely everything about this fetus looks normal and healthy, including the gastric pseudo-mass.

Eleanor sighs. "I know you told me not to worry. But when you had me come meet you in the office, I was scared. This doesn't seem like a big deal."

"It's not," I say. "I just needed a few minutes to be sure."

After they leave, I finally write my ultrasound report. "Gastric pseudo-mass, of no clinical significance, incidentally noted." In

Regular Person English that means, "I saw something, but I'm not worrying about it, and neither should you."

. . .

THE FIRST PURPOSE of Medical Language is to allow doctors to communicate better with ourselves and with each other; it helps create a shared basis for communication so that everybody knows which tendon we need to fix or why I'm running down the hallway to the operating room. It helps create an efficient communication for people who are doing the same job.

But as in any other language, any translation is also an interpretation. Moving words and feelings and information from Regular Person English into Medical Language does, by definition, introduce distance between those doctors and that regular person. Medical Language treats the human body as a problem to be solved, a collection of molecules and bundles of cells that can be understood and manipulated. That's what doctors are doing, so that's what the language needs to reflect. But that reflection can feel objectifying, arguably because it is.

Like other supposedly neutral languages, Medical Language—language theoretically invented to be standardized, neutral, unbiased—is thus very easily perceived as hostile. The very language that makes the care of the human body possible can at the same time make the people we are using it on feel like we don't even see them.

. . .

LONG AGO, IN the middle of a cold winter, I started taking a writing class online. I had graduated residency and was working as an attending. I finally had some time in my life to pursue this idea of creative writing that had nagged at me for years.

I never met my writing teacher, Mark, or any of the other students; we existed as a chat room at 8 p.m. on Monday nights. During one of those Monday nights, on the screen, Mark was making a point about a story I had submitted a few days earlier. He felt that my language was clear but also clinical and cold.

During this chat, he sent me his operative report from his brain surgery five years earlier. "It reminds me of this," he said. "And this report made me hate my surgeon; because it made me feel like he hated me."

Later, in an e-mail exchange, Mark told me that he had requested the operative summary of his benign brain surgery from five years earlier. He had requested it because he enjoys language and was looking forward to reading an account of an event that was important to him, an event in which he had taken part but had no awareness of. But after he read it, he wanted to walk up to his neurosurgeon and punch him in the mouth.

Mark read descriptions similar to this one:

> The head was turned to the left and rested on a doughnut. The scalp was shaved, and then prepped and draped in usual sterile fashion. Incisions were marked along a right frontotemporal craniotomy frontally and over the parietal boss; the incision was opened and carried down to the skull. Self-retaining retractor was placed. A bur hole was now fashioned with the perforator. This was widened with a 2-mm Kerrison punch.[3]

He read paragraphs describing the surgery, the dissection of his brain tissue and the removal of the mass. He read about rolling his body from side to side to optimize surgical approach; he read about the closings of his brain coverings and bone. He read about the fashioning of a bandage, the return to the postanesthesia care unit, and his return to consciousness. That return to consciousness, of course, is his only awake appearance in the whole story.

Mark told me that he read this with horror. It wasn't the use of the saw to open his skull or a hole puncher on his brain that felt violent. The shaving of the head, the sawing open of the forehead—none of that was what felt aggressive to him. It was the dispassionate way it was described; it was both very intimate and completely impersonal. It's not the cracking of the skull that bothered him; it's that the description of that act, an act that required Mark to trust the surgeon as he rarely trusted anyone previously, contained no acknowledgment that the skull held a brain and that this brain was the basis of a person's essence and intellect, and not just of any person, but of this person, this one wild and precious life.[4]

The operative report that Mark shared with me was, from a medical perspective, perfectly reasonable. It did what it was supposed to do, by which I mean, I could read it and understand what occurred during the surgery. The op report was even well written, by which I also mean that if I was a neurosurgeon, I could read the report and repeat the operation. But this was exactly the problem: to my writing teacher, it was reduction of his head to a collection of impersonal anatomic structures, and that felt like a rejection of his particular human self in a way that he found unbearable. The reason Mark hated this was because he could have been anyone, as though his surgeon thought of him as no one.

I know this feeling, because I've done it to myself. I forced the application of Medical Language to myself and then felt how little it made of my suffering. In my own first pregnancy, I was so careful never to say that there was a baby or even that there would be one. I called what was growing in my belly a "pregnancy" or a "fetus"; I asked my husband to do the same. I still don't know if he thought I was being crazy, but he knew it was important to me, and his general willingness to take me seriously is one of the reasons I married him.

This was the way my colleagues and supervisors spoke, because it reflected the reality we saw every day. We knew how terribly fine the line was between each day of pregnancy and a healthy baby. We knew, first hand, how just one bleed or one missed gene or one infection was the difference between this fetus and a healthy baby that would never be. I knew that most pregnancies ended well, but experientially, I had seen and touched and delivered all manner of terrible outcomes; that "most" felt far away.

I was trying so hard to be clinical, to be logical, to be fair, to treat myself as I treat my patients, because if I didn't, what did that say about the kind of doctor I was? But I was also so sick and so scared. I had nausea that wouldn't go away; I had the worry that comes from knowing intimately and experientially how many things could go wrong. I knew exactly how many steps stood between where I was at 12 weeks, at 14 weeks, at 20 weeks, and a live healthy baby; I knew how easily I could lose it all. I couldn't call it a baby because it wasn't yet, and I knew that maybe it would never be.

I used clinical language to describe my own body, even as I watched my life narrow to the minutes I would have to leave early in the morning so that I could throw up before I went into the office, to the trips to the bathroom to check for more bleeding, to the hours between nausea medications, to the days lost to side effects from those medications. Then one day, 23 weeks pregnant, I found myself in tears, kneeling on the bathroom floor, 14 hours into a 25-hour shift in the hospital, trying to get myself back to my patients on the labor floor. What the fuck was the point? I didn't want to be Medical Language pregnant; I wanted to be Regular Person pregnant. Using Medical Language about myself was too cruel. I didn't want a pregnancy; and I didn't want a fetus. I wanted a baby.

.   .   .

MEDICAL LANGUAGE DESCRIBES but distances; it creates the possibility for mechanization but also, then, for repairs. But Medical Language also has another function, as all language does: it signals. Whatever the words actually say, Medical Language is also a neon-lit marquee that says: this speaker is a medical professional who has undergone medical education. Using this specialized technical language highlights the differences between the person speaking it and a regular person in the same way that Military Language and Police Language and Academic Professor Language do.

In theory, the difference between speakers and nonspeakers of Medical Language could be of neutral value, but as with any language, that's almost never true. Speakers of Medical Language are often showing that they have more knowledge or more education; in many situations, those speakers hold more power. The use of Medical Language doesn't just create a void of misunderstanding; it draws a thick red line between the medical provider and the patient, creating distance between those two people at the very time that circumstances dictate that they work together.

Interestingly, this issue doesn't exist just between speakers of Medical Language and speakers of Regular Person. As with any language, Medical Language itself has dialects. One prime exam-

ple of this differential is the doctor-nurse divide. From almost
the beginning of these professions, nurses and doctors have been
speaking different kinds of Medical Language. From the outside
these appear to be minor linguistic differences, but very quickly
those differences can become a danger to patient safety. The language divide is not the only reason that nurse-doctor relations
have been complex and occasionally strained for as long as they've
existed, but the frequent absence of functional communication
language serves nobody well.

There are millions of examples highlighting this difference, litter-
ing the floors of ICUs and malpractice courts. Here's one example: a
37-year-old woman was admitted with very high blood pressure values.[5] Because the blood pressures were "reported to the MD" in the
emergency room, the nurse didn't report them to the doctor responsible for the inpatient floor. The nurse did note the patient's nausea and
pain and called the doctor overnight twice to get orders for antinausea medication and pain medication. The patient's blood pressures
remained high but were never transmitted to the overnight doctor
in numbers, so the physician never came to evaluate the patient. In
the morning, the patient was found unresponsive on the floor of her
room; she was pronounced dead after an unsuccessful resuscitation.
The diagnosis made after autopsy was of an aortic dissection—a
known complication of long periods of acute, uncontrolled elevated
blood pressure. The nurse said she told the doctor; the doctor said
he was never told the specific information that accurately represented
the level of concern.

I wish I could say that stories like this are rare, but they continue
to be commonplace. Long ago, as a second-year resident covering the
gynecology services overnight, I was covering two hospitals and three

services, including any patients in the emergency department and all the gynecology postoperative patients in the hospital. I had five pagers weighing down my scrub pants, and I was constantly hitching up and retying my waistband. In that age of numeric-only pagers and unreliable cell phones, I would get a page with a phone number and nothing else. There was no way to know if it was an emergency or something minor, so I constantly had to stop whatever I was doing and run to the nearest house phone. Most calls, that night and every night, were for simple things: an RN asking for a Tylenol order for a patient with a minor headache or a diet order for a postop patient for whom the day team had forgotten to change food preferences.

I called one nurse back, and she told me that a recent postoperative patient had a fever. This is not uncommon; many patients on their first day postsurgery will have a fever. We're all taught that the fever is rarely infectious; most real infections take several days to develop. Postop fevers are usually short-lived and don't require antibiotics. I had an actively bleeding patient in the emergency department, so I didn't ask the all-important question: "Do you need me to see the patient?" I didn't ask any follow-up questions at all, actually, given that I was in the middle of trying to stop some active bleeding and had at least one other pager beeping at me at the same time. I told the nurse that it was probably inflammatory, not infectious. I told her that I'd write her for some stuff and I got off the phone with the nurse. I quickly wrote a Tylenol order and for some IV hydration in the computer and ran to the next patient, the next page, the next bleed.

I didn't even think about the patient with the fever until 2 hours later when, on my way to the call room for a possible nap, I remembered that I hadn't yet seen her. Nobody had called me again, so I assumed she was fine and could wait until morning. But wait—had I heard a number on that fever? I didn't remember, and for some reason, I dragged myself back to the elevator and up to the postsurgical floor.

There I was appalled to find a patient with a fever—yes, a fever I had been told about. But I hadn't been told that she had a temperature of 104.1, much too high, and a heart rate of 130 beats per minute, despite the Tylenol and fluids. When I took her blood pressure, it was trending low—90/40, a possible sign of a patient who is about to crash from septic shock.

"Shit," I said. "Has she been like this the whole time? She needs antibiotics. She may need to be in the ICU."

"I called you about the fever!" the nurse said.

"But you didn't tell me how high!" I said "You didn't call me back when she didn't get better."

The nurse furiously replied, "Well, you told me it was nothing!"

"Because you didn't tell me any of this!"

It's true; I hadn't asked. I had assumed that a competent nurse would tell me any other abnormal vital signs—which is a reasonable expectation of a trained medical professional—but I also hadn't asked.

Some of this dysfunction can be attributed to history and education: for centuries, nursing education stressed the use of descriptive and subjective language, while doctors were taught to be directive and concrete, focusing on objective fact.

Nursing education taught this communication style to nurses in both positive ways ("paint the broad picture"; "pay attention to the things the patient doesn't say: how they're moving, how they're dressed") but also negative and disempowering ways ("it's not your job to diagnose"). In contrast, as discussed earlier, doctors are expressly taught language that focuses on the concrete and on getting to a diagnosis and a plan.

To honestly discuss this language difference, it is important to note that in the history of modern medicine, the vast majority of nurses have been women, and the vast majority of doctors have been men. (Even today, when half or more medical students are women, the overall number of practicing female doctors in the United States tops out at 34 percent, given the asymmetric differential from past decades.) Gender stereotypes have been baked right into the discipline of nursing from the beginning. When Florence Nightingale started to establish what we currently recognize as modern nursing in the nineteenth century,[6] her philosophy was that every woman was a nurse, and every woman who entered the nursing profession was only doing what came naturally to her.[7] Through much of the start of nursing as a profession, nursing schools were trained to be deferential to doctors, to adhere to routine, and to be caring toward the patient above all else. The caring quality of women was the ideal for all women; in nursing, this quality was seen as the reason that women could be responsible for hygiene, routine, and administration of medications, all "in faithful obedience to the physician's orders."[8] This caring, deferential persona was in stark contrast to the doctor and his masculine ideal: unsentimental, decisive, objective, distant, rational.

Though the language divide between doctors and nurses would seem to fit quite neatly within the "men are from Mars, women are from Venus" school of pop psychology, this divide ends up being an effective example of how this behavior is historical and taught rather than innate and necessary. Like pop psychology, the neat schema of different communication styles is not actually true or helpful in describing reality. Many studies in the literature debunk this gender-dichotomous view of the world.

One large study performed by Bobbi Carothers and Harry Reis

reviewed 13 studies of multiple physical and social criteria—including communication styles—in relation to gender.[9] The study showed that we are attracted to this strict dichotomy about gender communication; we love the idea that women say this and men say that. But the dichotomy falls apart under statistical scrutiny. For example, in their study (and in most of our lived experiences), it was relatively common for men to be empathetic and women to be good at math—characteristics that some research has associated with the other sex, says Carothers. "Sex is not nearly as confining a category as stereotypes and even some academic studies would have us believe," she added. In another interview, Reis said, "Clearly, it's not so much sex, but human character that causes difficulties."[10] As many of us already knew, no matter how strange and difficult to understand your doctor or nurse or boyfriend or mother might be, their gender is probably only a very small part of the problem.

All of this—Medical Language and the gendered roles it expresses—is, of course, in a constant state of change. After World War II, nursing education and work underwent a rapid and comprehensive professionalization.[11] Nursing began to become a serious vocation that required a large number of technical skills and scientific knowledge rather than just womanly skills and the ability to follow the doctor's orders. Women started training in universities and nursing schools, rather than solely at hospitals; degrees took longer, and women continued to work as nurses even after marriage. The discipline of nursing was no longer considered a set of female behaviors in a medical setting; it appropriately acknowledged the increasingly professional skill set and knowledge required to do this work in a complicated medical world.

The artificiality of this communication divide is interesting to explore as the gender assumption is violated more and more, with increasing numbers of female doctors and male nurses. Nurses used to be almost entirely women, and that balance has changed dramatically: in 1970, only 2.7 percent of nurses were men; that rose to 10 percent in 2013, and the proportion continues to rise.[12] In 1949, only 5.5 percent of entering medical students were women; by 1986, it was 36.4 percent; and most recently, it's been over 50 percent according to many studies.[13]

As those fields trend toward egalitarianism, what we start to note is that this language divide can be seen more as a reflection of the hierarchy within medicine: doctors as the highest rung of medical personnel have, of course, the fanciest words, the most definitive adjectives, the most medical of Medical Language to themselves.[14] And that hierarchy has ramifications: the literature is full of nurses being abused and being treated poorly; of surgeons throwing body parts or spewing expletives. All that is true and terribly unprofessional, and most medical schools have educational classes that try to address these problems.

But on occasion, the hierarchy exists in other, more unexpected directions. Seeing the language differences as a power differential is a more helpful structure for understanding the situation than gender is. Language can be used to denigrate people in different ways, reflecting that the power differential can be dependent on different strengths in different contexts. Sometimes the one being humiliated is a medical student or a medical trainee or even a fully credentialed doctor, new to this particular operating suite, who is on the lower end of the power and language scale. When we look at these languages as less a reflection of gender and more of power, the experiences that many of us have at work make a lot of sense.

For example, I've been on both sides of this kind of communication snafu many times; I've been both the dismisser and the dismissee. As a medical student, I asked a health aide—someone with just a few months of training—where to wash my hands. She sent me to the "dirty" sink and then laughed loudly because I didn't know that the dirty sink was only for equipment and not hands and sneered at me as I wandered around with my hands in the air. I had a scrub tech mock me and eject me from a surgery—not just once, but twice—because she didn't like how I stood at the operating table.

As an intern, I had my concerns about a patient dismissed by nurses who told me that, as an intern, I was just wasting everybody's time. This didn't happen just once or twice, but almost every night. Years later, when I was a fully credentialed attending in a new hospital, I had run-ins with nurses who had more power than I did and who used the language they had—language of administration, of malpractice—to push me toward doing a cesarean delivery that I didn't think was necessary.

And I'm sure I continue to do this, too, to use my language as a blunt instrument against patients and trainees. I've never thrown a gallbladder at my chief resident (a story I heard during my general surgery rotation; I was also told that the thrower became the head of the department a few years later). But I have denigrated a trainee's concerns about a patient with high blood pressure by reciting the ACOG criteria for hypertensive diseases of pregnancy at them; and I have made a patient cry because I told her that her gestational diabetes was a pathological process and that she needed to get with the treatment program. I have been beaten up by Medical Language, and I'm sure I've bludgeoned others with it.

WHOEVER THE PLAYERS are in twenty-first-century medicine, it seems clear that most of our problems communicating in Medical Language are taught to us during our training—and can be untaught. The time has come to do that unteaching, because the difference in Medical Language dialects has become counterproductive and unsafe in the modern world—or at least we've begun to notice what probably always was dangerous.

One of the main solutions to MD/RN language differences is the idea of the acronym SBAR. (It is, of course, so typical of Medical Language that the concept for making communication better would come with an acronym that's almost impossible to say.) SBAR stands for Situation Background Assessment Recommendation, and it's a way to standardize and construct a transfer of medical information.[15]

In the past, a nurse (which nurse? from where? I'm covering four floors and five different services) might call to tell me "I'm uncomfortable with a patient's heart rate," which, to a busy doctor, invites reassurance and a snooze button. With SBAR, the nurse would call and say: "This is Liz, nurse on the postpartum unit 5 South (the situation). Patient Smith is postop day zero from an uncomplicated cesarean and now has a persistent tachycardia. I've tried hydrating her, but it hasn't resolved (the background). I'm concerned about acute blood loss (the assessment); I'd like you to come see the patient right away; please also order a stat hematocrit, which I'll draw while you're on the way (the recommendation)." Bam. No reassurance; no snooze button. SBAR required Liz to think about what was important to tell me and what she wanted. But the payoff is that I know who Liz is; I know how worried she is; I know that she wants me to be on my way.

That's the concept, at least. In real life, SBAR does work, though it's awfully hard to implement. For many nurses, it means additional work to prepare for that phone conversation; to do some of the cognitive work before phoning the doctor, not process during it. SBAR also requires—and facilitates—a certain level of confidence from the speaker and a receptiveness in the listener, and in fact, this expectation, more than any actual format changes or word choices, is probably the largest part of why it works. But SBAR does work; it brings two professionals into the same language so that they can work together there.

. . .

MEDICAL LANGUAGE CREATES meaning and destroys closeness; it demands clarity and blurs nuance; it initiates healing and damages relationships, all at the same time. These powers affect its speakers, even when they're speaking plain English in a medical setting. Among the saddest examples are the words "I'm sorry."

In regular life, "I'm sorry" is one of the earliest phrases we learn: "Say sorry for taking your sister's toy. Say sorry for biting your brother. Say sorry for setting the kitchen on fire."

But "I'm sorry" is a complex phrase, even way back in childhood. It's a phrase that expresses sorrow but also regret and, along with those, some measure of blame and accountability. The double meaning of sorrow and blame makes "I'm sorry" an impossible phrase in Medical Language. Doctors often want to express sorrow, but not identify blame. Or perhaps the trail of accountability and guilt is too long and complicated for the simplistic reality of "I'm sorry." I'm sorry the cancer returned? I'm sorry the chemo didn't work? Or I'm sorry that we didn't operate earlier because I didn't pay enough attention to your pain? Or perhaps a bit of all of those?

This means that this earliest expression of sorrow is transformed for Medical Language speakers. It becomes laden and verboten; it is transformed into something useless. Doctors then become reluctant or even unable to say "I'm sorry" because it sounds like they did something wrong. But without "I'm sorry," how does a doctor start a conversation about terrible news? How does she express sympathy or even empathy? How does she let a patient grieve? And how does she grieve next to them?

. . .

ONE OF MY patients, Amanda Soldati, was young and quick; she spoke in choppy lilting sentences, with her mind always at the end of the sentence before her mouth was. She was so bright, always moving, hopping up on the bed as soon as I came into the room, wiggling her sneakered feet while talking. Amanda came to me after a tragedy the prior year; she had been pregnant and lost the pregnancy in second trimester after extremely preterm labor.

During her first visit for this pregnancy, her first pregnancy after her second-trimester loss, I talked with Amanda about all her options. The most invasive would be a surgical one; given her prior second-trimester miscarriage, she qualified as someone who might benefit from placing a stitch around her cervix, a procedure called a cerclage. At that first visit, I reviewed that similar outcomes were seen in pregnancies monitored by ultrasound; that is, we could be vigilant and wait and monitor her cervix. If her cervix started to shorten on ultrasound, then we would place a cerclage; but many women continued to have a normal cervix and normal pregnancy and avoid the procedure altogether. Amanda paced the room a bit but ultimately decided that watchful waiting seemed reasonable; and wouldn't it be nice to avoid a surgery and all the associated risks?

Three weeks later, I got a call from the ultrasound unit: Amanda's cervix was short; not dangerously so, but definitely no longer normal. I called Amanda on the phone; we talked about the risks and benefits of the cerclage at this point. It wasn't, even now, a simple decision; one of the risks of surgery includes the possible puncture of the amniotic membranes by the surgery itself, which would lead to the loss of pregnancy. But Amanda definitely wanted the cerclage now; she told me she didn't want to waste any more time.

The next day, I took Amanda to the operating room. I placed her cerclage myself. The procedure was uncomplicated and short; I showed her a wiggling fetus on ultrasound in the recovery room. She went home later that day with a plan to see me in a week.

Six days later, Amanda returned, not to clinic but to the hospital in the middle of the night. She was writhing in pain as her uterus contracted against her stitched cervix. Amanda's cervix started to tear around the cerclage, and she started to bleed heavily. The overnight team removed her cerclage, and Amanda delivered less than an hour later. The fetus, at 22 weeks, did not survive.

I saw Amanda the next day on the gynecology floor. She had asked to be taken away from the regular postpartum floor for her recovery; she didn't want to hear the babies crying. She knew to ask for this, of course, because she had been through it before.

When I came in, Amanda was lying wordless in the bed. Her eyes were open and she nodded to me, but she was pale and still, so unlike her usual self. I saw her sneakers and jeans stuffed into a clear bag, dumped on the windowsill. I dragged a chair from the hallway into her room and thought about what I wanted to say.

I wanted to say, "I'm sorry. God, I'm so sorry. I'm sorry we didn't place the cerclage earlier in the pregnancy. I'm sorry I placed the cerclage at all. I'm sorry that you bled because of the surgery I did, the surgery that didn't work. I'm sorry that my team took out the cerclage. I'm sorry about all of this."

All of that was true, but there were more complicated truths, too: that we didn't know then what we knew now; that we had made good decisions—decisions together—that I could still stand by. I was grieving but not regretful; I was sad, but not guilty.

And yet, so much sorrow in that room. So much care and surgery and pain and bleeding, and here she was, with none of what we worked for, none of what she wanted, and nothing that she deserved. How do you say that truth in any language?

.   .   .

THERE'S A LARGE body of medical literature about teaching doctors how to "break bad news," how to communicate with patients about bad things that happened—in other words, how to translate Medical Language into Regular Person under the worst circumstances. Breaking bad news is one of the most stressful things that doctors do; some studies show that having to discuss a failed resuscitation— having to tell a family that we lost their loved one—is something that doctors feel less competent at than the complex resuscitation itself.[16] Many doctors don't discuss these bad events; or they communicate them in ways that are not helpful, that are perceived as distant or emotionless, that lead to anger, hostility, or even legal action. For the doctor, the difficulty of this kind of communication leads to profound emotional exhaustion; over time, that leads to stress and ulti-mately burnout. More than we'd like, physicians leave their field, the field they trained for decades to work in. On a personal level this can be a disaster; on a public health level, this burnout can lead to medi-cal personnel shortages and becomes a catastrophe.

Thus, we see a growing effort to teach doctors how to break bad news, with increasing educational and communication resources devoted to the idea that this skill is as important to being a capable, long-lived doctor as the correct handling of a scalpel or knowledge of new medications. One of the most important things that these skill lessons have taught me is how to handle the thorny problem of "I'm sorry." It feels like it must be semantics, it's that simple, but it works, and here is what it is. Instead of saying "I'm sorry," you say, "I wish things were different."

That phrase "I wish" is similar to "I'm sorry" in its simple roots, its childhood origins. It dissects out the sorrow, the grief, and leaves behind the blame. The doctor can wish for a different universe, one where this terrible thing had never happened; one where the surgery went well, or where the cancer didn't return, or where the pregnancy developed normally. "I wish" calls for a different universe to come into being; the phrase itself alludes to the fact that we cannot travel there. But the phrase also allows for the yearning we feel for that universe and the sorrow we feel that we can't get there.

Instead of being stuck in Medical Language, across a locked door from someone who speaks Regular Person Language, the doctor can say, "Something terrible has happened, and I so very much wish it hadn't. I wish this world were different. I wish today were different. I wish this hadn't happened."

And that unlocks the door between us.

. . .

THAT DAY, IN the dim room on the gynecology floor of the hospital, I finished dragging my chair into her room, toward the head of
her bed. I sat down, and I was quiet for a moment. For a long time,
Amanda didn't talk, and then she did. She told me how sad she was
and how horrible it had been and how everything was lost and how
nothing would ever be right. I listened for a long time.

When she was done, I didn't have much to add. I said the only
thing I could think to say: "I wish this hadn't happened. I'm so sad
that we're here now." It was inadequate, but it was true.

THIRD TRIMESTER

5.

Periviable Birth

A Necessary Story

All medical experiences, but especially labor and delivery, need to be good stories. I don't mean that they need to be interesting or suspenseful. In some ways, it's the opposite: the story of good medical care is one that is sturdy and well constructed and, quite often, boring. Good care is a series of observations that leads logically to a series of choices that lead, in turn, to an understandable course of action. In satisfactory medical practice, all of these events should march steadily, one after another to a predictable end.

For example, a patient with a cough and fever and an X-ray showing signs of pneumonia should get antibiotics. Antibiotics given without the X-ray or the cough would be malpractice; and infection without antibiotics may be negligence. The story must cohere, or the doctors in the story have not done their job.

The vast majority of the time, the narrative of a labor and delivery is short and ends in joy: labor, delivery, Apgar score 9 and 9, happy outcome. But sometimes, labor and delivery is a place of terrible choices, choices that only the woman at the center can make. This means that this woman needs to choose her own terrible adventure, even while she's going through it, because if she doesn't make those choices, then someone else will write her story instead.

· · ·

SOME OF US are calling it a baby. Some of us are calling it a fetus. Some of us are calling it "it," though we catch ourselves when we do. None of us feel good about any of this.

We're all talking to Annie Riley but really to her whole family. She's pregnant, 23 weeks and 0 days by our best estimates. Until yesterday, she was having a normal, uncomplicated pregnancy. Then yesterday, when she was running errands, her water broke. She came to see us, and while being evaluated, she became uncomfortable. Now she's in labor. We are trying to stop the labor, this complicated process by which our body works to eject the contents of the uterus. Our treatments for this situation are old and not terribly effective. Right now it looks very much like she will be delivering within the next few hours or days.

So we're in her room, talking and talking about the pregnancy, about the fetus, about the baby. Is it a baby or a fetus? That's the thing, really, the crux of the matter. We need her to tell us.

Here is her limited menu of options:

- Option A, the story of a miscarriage. In this story, the pregnancy is a fetus. It is less than 24 weeks. The rate of survival at this gestational age is very low. Those infants that have survived are overwhelmingly affected by the sequelae of their extreme prematurity, including blindness, lung problems, and cerebral palsy. The chance of getting a child out of this process is small; the chance of getting a healthy child is vanishingly small. If she chooses this story of miscarriage, we will allow the fetus to be born; we will not torture it with tubes and sharp stings. We will offer "comfort care" and make sure it is warm and place it on Annie's chest for as long as it stays in this world with us.

- Option B, the story of an extremely preterm birth, not a miscarriage. In story B, the pregnancy is a baby. A baby will be born, and we will fight for its life. We will place tubes and lines in its tiny translucent body. We will bring to bear all the wisdom and knowledge, all the science and computers, everything we have. It likely won't be enough. The baby might still die; the baby will probably still die. It if lives, it will probably be impaired, somewhere between moderately and severely so.

Annie has to pick a story; we are all very insistent that she has to pick a story, as soon as possible. Why? Because if it's story B, we will start to do things to her, and some of those things are not very nice. We will give her strong medications to try to offer the baby some narrow advantage when it's born; we will strap her to the bed and vigilantly monitor the heart rate of the baby. We will swarm in and out of the room, touch her and examine her and poke her for blood tests. We will consider offering her an emergent cesarean delivery, with all the risks entailed by urgent major abdominal surgery. The kind of cesarean delivery we will offer her will, by virtue of the anatomy available to us at 23 weeks gestation, be a vertical uterine incision, which will compromise all of her future pregnancies and deliveries. We will do that even though the chance of this baby leaving the operating room alive is less than 30 percent.[1]

For story A, we won't do any of it. We will not even listen to the fetal heart rate because we wouldn't do anything differently—we don't do major abdominal surgery and risk a woman's health if it's not going to change an outcome. We will make the room quiet and peaceful; we will try to make sure she has one stable provider and a nurse who knows her and who is good at this kind of situation. We will hang a picture of a leaf with a teardrop on the door so that all members of the staff know that a loss is occurring in this room. When the delivery happens, we will give the family time. We will help them take pictures and start a memory box. We will mourn.

Until Annie makes her choice, her providers are so very uncomfortable. Because what is good care in story A is malpractice in story B, and vice versa. How can we care for this patient until she tells us what care is?

.   .   .

YOU KNOW, I'VE done this for a reasonably long time now. And for the first part of that time, I had to learn how the medical story is constructed. This is most of what you spend the second half of medical school doing, learning how to tell the story. Once upon a time there was abdominal pain with the right lower quadrant tenderness and the elevated white blood cell count. It's a story called appendicitis, and it needs to end in the operating room, just as surely as the knight must slay the dragon; if it doesn't, you need to explain why.

Once upon a time there was a woman who was pregnant, and she went into preterm labor with a baby who was resuscitated; it's a sad story. Once upon a time, there was a woman who was pregnant, and she had a 23-week miscarriage; it's also a sad story.

But what we're not good at—as patients but also as medical providers—is seeing how everything is more than one story. It can be read this way or that; sometimes it needs to be read this way and then changed. Storytellers can make mistakes, after all.

During the first part of our medical education, we learn to tell the story. Later in our medical education, we learn to let go halfway through and sometimes tell a different story.

. . .

NORA SALMAN HAD only one prenatal care visit with our hospital, just this week, at 35 weeks pregnant. She did have first-trimester labs done somewhere else; from her purse, she produced a wadded-up purple "pregnancy passport" that had a negative HIV test scribbled on her 12-week visit. But then she had a second HIV test done just last week, on her first visit to our hospital. This is our protocol for patients in their third trimester. Nora's third-trimester HIV test was positive.

Third-trimester HIV is a risk for her, but also a risk for her baby. The baby can get the virus during labor and delivery and live with it its whole life. Or we can prevent that, right now.

The initial HIV test at the time we took care of Nora was a tricky one; it was known to be falsely positive a large portion of the time. Back then, this false-positive result was frequent enough that it didn't generate an official report because it was only a partial result. What it did generate was a reflex test, called a Western blot, a more precise protein assay to tell us whether the result was real or not.

When Nora came into labor and delivery, her Western blot was still pending, currently in process on the countertop of some anonymous lab. For right now, there's the positive partial HIV test in our hand and a woman in labor in front of us.

If Nora truly had uncontrolled HIV, our doctors could have offered her a cesarean to minimize transmission to the baby. But they've got that crumpled purple paper from first trimester and her very clear protestation that she hasn't had any new sexual partners since then and that her partner hasn't either. Nora is 100 percent sure she doesn't have HIV; no, 1,000 percent sure.

The overnight team doesn't recommend a cesarean; major surgery based on a probable false positive seems extreme. But they do want to do something relatively low-risk, something that can offer the newborn protection from lifelong HIV. They start antiviral medications during labor. Antiviral HIV medications, like zidovudine, can prevent transmission to the neonate during labor and delivery. The plan is to stop the meds if her result returns negative. That's the plan.

Morning comes. Nora is still pregnant. I join the team on the labor and delivery floor, rounding on the high-risk patients. I check the computer; the Western blot has a result. It is, as we have all hoped, negative. Negative! I crow. That's wonderful. But then I look closer; that result has been back since 3 a.m. Why is she still on the zidovudine? The team hems and haws. We just ... the night team was too busy to discuss it. The day team wasn't sure. We wanted to talk it over. We wanted to be sure, you know?

I do know. Once you have a label, it's very hard to let go of it. Once you have a story, it's very difficult to change to another narrative. Even if the story is false; even if you can point to digits on the computer screen that say that this story is not true. Still, the absence of action—the not treating of this patient—comes hard, too hard for a team that entered with one reality and exited with another, just wanting to do the right thing and not sure enough to know what the "right thing" is. The patient was already exposed to the risks of the medication, right? So what's another dose or two until we make sure that everyone agrees that this is the new truth?

Let's turn off the ZDV, I say. Everyone laughs but nobody moves. In the end, I have to write the order myself; I ask the nurse if she wants me to push the off button on the IV pump, but she tells me that now I'm being silly.

"Am I?" I say.

. . .

ONCE UPON A time, there was a woman with HIV. She came to us to have a baby, and we kept that baby healthy by giving large doses of intravenous medications. We were heroes, and we won.

That is a story, but is it this woman's story, today? No. The story changed, but we kept rolling forward, handicapped by our medical narrative, by the story we were telling. We keep our sword out, chopping at the dragon who has long ago left the building or perhaps never existed at all.

If we get better at this, maybe we can figure that story out more accurately. Maybe we can figure out how to look at the dragon in the story. Are you the real enemy? Do we need to have this fight?

. . .

ANOTHER DAY, ANOTHER labor floor.

Nadia Triggs is sad. She has known this day was coming; for the most part, she chose it. She is laboring away in a labor room in the corner, in comfort and in quiet, since her epidural was placed several hours ago.

Nadia is sad because there is something so deeply wrong with her fetus, wrong in a way that means it won't live long with us. When we see the fetus on ultrasound, we can see right away the bell-shaped curve of the chest, tighter than the abdomen; the heart taking up a huge portion of a too-small chest cavity; the bones shaped in a curved embrace, too tight; no room for lungs to develop, and so none have.

The fetus is doing all right for now, in its small fishlike space where oxygen comes from the umbilical cord, where it doesn't need lungs. But when it gets out here, to us, it will need to breathe air through the mouth and nose and through the lungs it does not have. And so, we have told her, the baby will die.

This is the account Nadia was told, by one wise man and then another wise woman, as we all struggled to understand what we saw inside her. It's the story I read in her record; it's the story she told me when she came into the hospital to have her labor started. She had already decided with those wise doctors that her labor would be one during which we would not monitor the fetus, since if it showed distress, none of us were willing to perform a cesarean delivery to deliver a baby that would not live, no matter how quickly and well we would act. Better not to look, the story goes, like many ancient stories before; you turn to salt, or worse.

But Nadia, laboring away in comfort and in quiet, now wants to look. She calls and asks to speak to me, and when I come in, she asks, "Can I listen to the baby's heart?" Her nurse stands by, uncomfortable. *This was not the plan.*

And I say, "Well, yes, of course. Yes. Of course. But can I remind you of the story we told each other? We talked about how if we watch the fetal heart rate go up and down and then go down and down and down, that's hard. That feels risky. Because my training—and the nurse's training, all of our training—is to rush you to the operating room and get the baby out. But," I say gently, "Getting the baby out fast, that's not relevant here. I wish it were different, but there's no surgery I can do, no matter how fast or how well, that can save this baby. And to watch the heart rate go down and down and down to zero—that's hard on you and hard on all the people taking care of you who have trained all their lives to prevent that. We might even, foolishly, forget who you are and do what we generally do. Risk to you, for no good reason, etcetera."

"I know all that," Nadia says. "But . . . it's just. I want to know if the baby is dead inside of me. I know we won't do anything differently. I just . . . I just want to know."

And I understand, finally. Inside this nightmare that she didn't know could exist of a malformed fetus who can breathe like a fish but not like a human, there is a worse nightmare. It's the nightmare of delivering a dead baby. And inside that nightmare is an even worse one—delivering a baby and not knowing that it is dead. We are three levels deep in a story she doesn't want to be in.

And I can take her one level back. She can live in just two nightmares.

I say, "What would you like? What if we checked every 20 minutes? Just a brief check, a few times every hour? We can do that."

"Yes," Nadia says and sighs with relief. "That is what I want."

We check every 20 minutes. There is always a heart rate, low but normal in the 120s. I will never know if there was distress during the labor, but the baby is born a few hours later, alive. Pediatrics is there; they assess the baby briefly, and there's not much they can do. They give the baby to the mother to have on her chest, to be with each other for as long as they have together.

TERM PREGNANCY

6.

Trial of Labor after Cesarean

Accept and Reject Intervention

At 2 a.m. on a Friday, she finally agreed to a cesarean.

Sarah Pasternak had been on the labor floor for 2 days—that was Wednesday, though it was hard to remember—after her early prenatal appointment that morning showed high blood pressure. She had protein on her urine dip at the office, and along with that blood pressure, she immediately met criteria for preeclampsia, a serious disease that can affect late pregnancy. Preeclampsia can be mild; but historically, it is also one of the reasons that women get sick and even die in pregnancy. The only cure for preeclampsia is delivery.

On that Wednesday morning, Sarah was already 39 weeks pregnant, so the decision to induce wasn't something the doctors argued over. Sarah's plan on that Wednesday morning had been a bagel with cream cheese on the way to work from the doctor's office; she never got that bagel, and by the time the nurse ushered her into a labor room at the hospital, the plan for breakfast, like most of her plans, was swept aside.

Sarah was brought to the labor room, where her husband joined her. IV lines were put in and labs were drawn; her cervix was checked and found to be 2 centimeters dilated. Sarah wanted to move around, but she was being put on magnesium to keep the preeclampsia from giving her seizures. The magnesium made her groggy and bleary-eyed, and the nurse told her it would be dangerous for her to be off the fetal monitor, so she ended up staying in bed. After 12 hours and multiple attempts at making her cervix softer, the oxytocin—a medicine meant to start contractions and open the cervix—was started.

Sarah's initial plan had been to try a medication-free childbirth. But 18 hours into the process, she was still 2 centimeters dilated despite hours of painful contractions; she asked for an epidural. That was Thursday, in the wee hours of the morning. Sarah slept, but people kept coming in and increasing the oxytocin. Sometimes they would examine her cervix, then sigh and shake their heads. She became 4 centimeters dilated but then was still 4 centimeters hours later. At some point—maybe it was Thursday, late morning?—someone used a hook to break her bag of waters. They didn't ask or warn her; they just did it.

By 6 p.m. Thursday, she was still 4 centimeters dilated. A new doctor came in, the Thursday evening shift, and told Sarah she should have a cesarean. Sarah's husband sat up, rumpled, in the bed by the window and didn't say anything. Sarah said no and started to cry.

By 1 a.m., the baby's heart rate was going up and wasn't coming down. Still 4 centimeters. The doctor told Sarah that she was likely on the way to an infection, given that her bag of waters was broken ("Broken by you people!" Sarah screamed, but only to herself). The doctor said, "I'm worried about the baby." The doctor recommended a cesarean again. Sarah was tired and hungry and confused and most of all scared. Sarah stopped saying no. She signed the paper they put in front of her. That was at 2 a.m. on Friday.

At 2:30 a.m., they took her to the operating room. They tugged at her and pulled and told her that what she was feeling wasn't pain, just pressure, but she couldn't help but scream a little anyway because it felt like pain has always felt like. And finally, after all that, a wail. The baby.

The next few days were blurry and awful: pain at her incision, dizziness and nausea from the pain meds; even sitting up to breastfeed was a two-person project. She felt sadness, and anger, too, murkily directed at the doctor, at the hospital, at her body; anger at her baby mixed in with disappointment, which wasn't any less strong 5 days postop when she visited the chirpy midwife who removed her staples.

Three years later, that baby is a healthy toddler. Sarah is physically recovered, mostly. She almost never cries about that Friday night anymore. She and her husband still use the hospital's name as a curse word; it works well as a synonym for "shit."

Sarah is pregnant again. She's looking for prenatal care. And she's friends with me, a high-risk obstetrician, so she calls me. She says, "I want whatever is the opposite of what we did the first time. I'm considering going into labor in a birthing center, or a home birth, or possibly just wandering into a forest and coming out when we're done." She's joking, but only mostly.

· · ·

I WANT TO start by saying that cesarean deliveries are a goddamn gift. To have a tool to get a baby out safely, quickly, and without killing the woman is a recent invention; women have had to fight for this tool, and I am grateful to be able to offer it when appropriate and necessary.

I also want to say that Sarah had a terrible experience, one that remains painful to her and caused trauma to her and to her young family. That is all true, and deeply regrettable, and wrong. And yet, for clarity's sake, I need to point something out: medically speaking, none of the decisions made during her treatment were technically incorrect. Would I have done the same had I been her doctor? I'd like to think I'd have explained more or been warmer or had her participate in the decision-making in a way that felt less traumatic. But the medical answer is that I would've made most of those same labor management decisions, and in fact, I can tell you that I have, dozens of times.

Let's look at this experience and the surgery that's at the heart of it. I'm going to use the terminology *cesarean delivery* or *cesarean birth* rather than *cesarean section*, because although it's a surgery, in the larger context of the life of a woman, it's also (and usually primarily) a birth, and not recognizing that is probably part of what creates the trauma. The occurrence of the urgent cesarean delivery already represents a trauma for many women—a failure, a mix of regret and blame that isn't associated with other surgeries. Few people have such complicated emotional landscapes surrounding their appendectomies. Birth is a life cycle event, and a complicated one; add an undesired surgery to that, and it becomes almost impossible to navigate.

Before the twentieth century, cesarean delivery was a rarity because it was also often fatal. By the second half of the nineteenth century, the adoption of antiseptic techniques, the move of birth from the home to hospital, and the advent of obstetric anesthesia meant that cesarean delivery became safer. But through the early part of the twentieth century, cesarean deliveries were rare: less than

2 percent of all deliveries in the United States in 1916 were surgical, likely because cesarean deliveries were still very dangerous; and 1933 statistics report a cesarean-related maternal mortality rate of 4 to 16 percent when looking at some of the best U.S. hospitals.[1]

In the early twentieth century, improvement in cesarean delivery safety came with a linear increase in the performance of cesarean delivery. Sometime in the late 1990s, the rate began to rocket upward, increasing exponentially.[2] Studies of that increase have noted that there was an increase both in first-time (or, as they are called in the medical literature, "primary") cesarean deliveries and in repeat cesarean deliveries. Put another way, almost half of the increase in overall cesarean births was related to a decrease in women successfully attempting a vaginal birth after cesarean (VBAC), also known as a trial of labor after cesarean (TOLAC).

This unsettling rise in cesarean delivery rate in the late twentieth and early twenty-first century means that currently, almost a third of all babies are now born by cesarean delivery, a statistic unthinkable 100 years ago. That unthinkable number describes our reality, despite the fact that the majority of both women and doctors want it to go down.

It's understandable that women (and most often, their doctors) would want to avoid cesarean deliveries. Even if the cesarean delivery wasn't a horrific experience, these surgeries are generally less safe than a vaginal delivery and can lead to future complications in this pregnancy and the next.[3] Most data show increasing complications for both women undergoing the surgery and babies born by surgery, compared with uncomplicated vaginal delivery. (Risks are higher in a complicated vaginal delivery; the trick, of course, is knowing who's going to have which.)

Here's the kicker: though I wish it weren't true, not all those cesarean deliveries are necessary. Some doctors don't do them for the right reasons. Sometimes those wrong reasons are systemic problems that have little to do with any individual doctor's desire to practice good medicine. For example, U.S. malpractice law generally makes it harder to defend not doing a cesarean than to defend doing one for the wrong reasons.[4] Even if an individual provider is aware of and resists this pressure, the overarching culture makes it awfully hard to sustain that level of practice. Other systemic contributors to increased cesarean rates include the perceived safety and control inherent in surgical birth (which is not true, but some women request cesareans for this reason). Additionally, our assumption of small family size may lead us to undervalue the complications that arise from repeated cesareans, since the assumption is that women will only need about two surgeries.

Finally, there are the cesarean deliveries that are done for terrible reasons. People joke about the obstetrician performing a cesarean because they want to get to their golf game or back to their Botox practice. I don't think that happens often; I've never met anyone who talked or practiced in such a way, although of course it's impossible to know for sure.

But we do have good data showing that when doctors are recompensed based on delivery rather than shift work, their cesarean rates go up.[5] That is, even if it's subconscious, the financial incentive to deliver all their patients themselves leads to a push that means the doctors will try to control that delivery in the most powerful way they have, by calling for a cesarean. This is why many large hospitals have transitioned to shift work. Although there are attendant frustrations, including my frustrated patients who want their own doctor, the truth is that data show that when we have shifts—when I go home at 8 a.m. regardless of whether the patient is still pregnant—we have better outcomes. For one thing, tired, distracted doctors are not trying to work endless hours. Second, it means that those doctors are no longer asked to be in two places at once—for example, monitoring a complicated labor course while attending to a busy clinic. Third, the doctors who work shifts have no incentive not to wait; they have every incentive toward patience. And patience is what most labors usually need to be successful and avoid cesarean deliveries.

Thus, for reasons good, bad, and deeply awful, cesarean deliveries in the United States are often overperformed. The secret to lowering the cesarean delivery rate is twofold: one, avoiding that first cesarean, and two, giving women who have had a cesarean a way out: the option to try a vaginal birth after cesarean (VBAC). As mentioned earlier, this is also known as a trial of labor after cesarean (TOLAC). TOLAC is the exit ramp from a lifetime of surgical births.

.   .   .

FROM THE MOMENT women began to survive cesarean deliveries in the early 1900s, there was interest in how to manage their next delivery. In Europe, TOLAC was considered an acceptable risk, but in the United States, different thinking prevailed: TOLAC was considered unsafe. This meant that it was very rare: in a 1968 study, more than 80 percent of New York City physicians thought that they would never consider TOLAC a safe action. It's not surprising, then, that 99 percent of patients with a previous cesarean delivery were delivered by an elective repeat cesarean delivery in American hospitals as late as 1974.[6]

Over time, the medical community's thinking about TOLAC has changed. As in many other arenas, there's been a move toward increased patient autonomy and shared decision-making. There's also the ugly truth that cesarean deliveries have risks that extend far beyond this pregnancy: a woman who has multiple cesareans may end up with anatomy so changed by scar tissue that each surgery becomes more and more dangerous and can ultimately limit her family size.

Then there's the very real increase of placenta accreta spectrum. With the increase in the cesarean rate, we are seeing more and more of these placentas: placenta accreta and increta and percreta. In the area of the uterus where the uterus has healed, the signals that tell a placenta to stop here, to implant only this far and no farther, are more likely to be compromised. Especially when there are multiple scars, a placenta can invade into or through the wall of a uterus, attaching firmly and refusing to let go. This is called a placenta accreta if it attaches past the lining of the uterus and into the muscle; a placenta increta if it's well into the thickness of the uterine muscle; and a placenta percreta if it burrows through the uterus and into adjacent structures: bladder, bowel, blood vessels.

Invasive placental disease is more likely to occur in a uterus with a scar, and the risk increases with the number of scars that have been placed in that uterus. It turns out that pregnancy isn't a benign growth; it needs to be a bilateral agreement between a woman's body and a developing embryo. Without limits, the pregnancy will continue to grow, to take and overtake. It doesn't take what it needs; it takes everything it can get.

If a woman has a placenta accreta, increta, or percreta, then that woman can hemorrhage—quickly and massively—during attempted removal of the placenta. In these situations, a hysterectomy usually has to be performed, often accompanied by massive blood loss and equally massive transfusion. If we know about the invasive placenta before delivery, late preterm delivery is recommended: planned, safe, timed to happen before a woman comes to us in labor or already bleeding. Even so, as recently as 2002, the maternal mortality rate was reported to be as high as 5 to 7 percent.[7] That is, of course, the worst-case scenario (see Chapter 10). But even the best-case scenario is a woman who has undergone major surgery, suffered dramatic bleeding, received enormous amounts of transfusion, lost the ability to carry a pregnancy, and has ended up in the ICU with a premature baby.

The rising cesarean delivery rate of the last decades was thus followed closely by a rise in occurrences of placenta accreta spectrum. In 1970, the rate of placenta accreta spectrum was 1 in approximately 4,000 patients; in the years 1980–2002, it was around 1 in 2,500 patients. The most recent data place the risk at 1 in 533 patients—almost a 10-fold increase over one generation.[8]

Current guidelines about TOLAC include the need for a thorough discussion of the risks and benefits of TOLAC compared with the risks and benefits of repeated cesarean delivery. That discussion needs to include ramifications not just for this pregnancy, but also for all the pregnancies a woman might want in the future. Those guidelines tell providers to offer women with one prior cesarean delivery a choice: proceed to repeat cesarean delivery or take the option of TOLAC.

.   .   .

EVEN THOUGH THOSE are technically the choices, a lot of women can't actually opt for TOLAC even if they want to. To safely offer

TOLAC deliveries, those same ACOG guidelines that advocate that patients be permitted to make a well-informed choice also recommended in 1998–99 that a hospital be able to provide an emergent cesarean "immediately," generally interpreted as within 30 minutes.[9] That capability requires a bunch of really expensive commitments and a lot of highly trained personnel, including 24/7 anesthesia coverage either in-house or very close by, as well as obstetrics attending physicians constantly on the labor floor. These were the ACOG recommendations, despite research showing that this level of resource use would be impossible to sustain for many small hospitals and editorials pointing out that other labor risks of similar magnitude (for example, a prolapsed cord) were tolerated regularly.[10] Rural hospitals serving large areas with a small population often can't muster that kind of coverage, which means that they often make the decision not to allow TOLAC at their sites. For women in large swathes of the country, this means that the one hospital in their area won't offer TOLAC, and there's often no other option within a 6-hour drive.[11] They end up with a repeat cesarean because their theoretical choice, unsupported by real resources, remained imaginary.

Almost immediately after the 1998–99 ACOG guidelines on TOLAC were published, the U.S. TOLAC rates crashed. Over a few years, the rate dropped from approximately 25 percent to less than 10 percent.[12] Most of that TOLAC loss was borne by rural America. In one study, TOLAC rates in rural Maine fell by more than half, from 30 percent in 1998 to less than 13 percent in 2001, and the most commonly cited reason was the inability of the hospital to meet with ACOG recommendations for the provision of labor after cesarean.[13] More recently, likely as a result of this dramatic change and the accompanying increase of placenta accreta cases, with all their morbidities, ACOG guidelines have utilized slightly more nuanced language as an attempt to reduce the burden on these hospitals.[14]

Despite those changes, the unavailability of TOLAC throughout many rural areas remains problematic. I talked to Andrea Greiner, a maternal-fetal medicine specialist in Iowa City. She said, "We have women who drive 3 or 4 hours so they can have a trial of labor after cesarean. That is challenging during Iowa winters." She points out that in the rural hospitals, "Family medicine doctors deliver babies, and the general surgeons [rather than OBGYN surgeons] do the c-sections; neither of them are in the hospital 24/7." This has led to some women finding that they have to move to the big city near the time of their birth to allow for TOLAC; others labor at home or while driving long distances, unmonitored. Still others have chosen to leave the medical system altogether and pursue a home birth, counter to ACOG recommendations about TOLAC at home, and Dr. Greiner has seen terrible complications from those cases as well (see Chapter 9).

Why has TOLAC been so tightly regulated? Why do hospitals get so nervous that they shut this service down entirely? Because 99 percent of the time, things go fine—or at least they go wrong in the usual ways. Most of the time the baby is born vaginally; sometimes a repeat cesarean delivery is needed, but 99 percent of the time, nothing horrendous happens.

But approximately 1 percent of the time, something horrendous does happen. That horrendous event is called uterine rupture; it's when the scar on the uterus, weaker than the surrounding unscarred muscle, breaks open. When the uterus ruptures, the uterus bleeds; this can be dangerous for the pregnant woman. But depending on luck, it's even more dangerous for the baby: if the rupture is near or under where the placenta is attached to the uterine wall, the baby can bleed and will also have less functional connection to the maternal oxygen it needs every minute.

In most studies, uterine rupture happens approximately 1 percent of the time. And 1 percent of the time is not the same as never.

. . .

JANE LUCAS COMES in to triage at 9 p.m. to get checked for contractions; her first baby had been breech, and she had undergone a cesarean delivery prior to labor, so this is a whole new experience for her. She is young and cheerful, excited for this baby to join her 3-year-old at home. She's been counseled about TOLAC several times and knows the numbers better than I do. Jane wants a big family, so avoiding another cesarean is a real priority for her: She wants to have at least five kids. Maybe more! A basketball team? A soccer team? Maybe a football team. I tell her that I'm from a big family, but only about half of us are remotely athletic; we joke that every team needs a manager. Between these conversations, we have Jane sign all our forms, including the consent for an emergent cesarean delivery if needed.

Jane is at 4 centimeters and the baby is low, with the fetal head right between her pelvic bones at 0 station. She's not in a lot of pain, but her cervical exam is more dilated than it was earlier in the day, when she was seen in clinic. Given that she's attempting TOLAC, we decide it would be best to admit her. I counsel her that she doesn't have to have an epidural but that I do like to offer it early in these situations: aside from pain control, it has the nice side benefit of giving our team a safe way to do surgery without her having to go to sleep if the TOLAC doesn't go well. Jane cheerfully agrees: "I've never been a huge fan of pain, anyway," she says.

She gets her epidural at around 1 a.m. and settles into bed; I examine her and she's now 6 centimeters. Her labor is progressing beautifully, and I relax a bit. Research shows that this is the best possible scenario for a VBAC; natural spontaneous labor offers the lowest risk for uterine rupture and the highest probability of successful vaginal birth.

But at 4 a.m., there's something on the monitor that doesn't look quite right. The residents call me, and I run downstairs; just a minute ago, the baby's heart started beating at a higher rate, abnormally high. Is Jane developing a fever? Is she dehydrated? I walk into the room, and as I do, I hear the baby's heart rate go from too high to too low, bump bump bump down the stairs, from 180 all the way down to the 60s. This is much more concerning; a baby can't live for long with a heart rate in the 60s.

We quickly do our usual maneuvers: turn the patient to give the baby more of the maternal circulation; put on an oxygen mask; open up her IV line to give her more fluid. Still 60s; we're now 2 minutes into this low heart rate. I quickly do a cervical exam to see what's going on. Now 4 centimeters; wasn't she 6 before? And that baby's head is floating, high in the pelvis, not even really in the pelvis anymore. That's not right. None of this is right. She's going backward in labor. Shit.

In that moment, I realize that labor is reversing because the scar from Jane's prior cesarean has blown open inside her belly. The baby is no longer being held down by the uterus because there's no uterus behind it anymore. She has a uterine rupture.

I yell out "Stat section; uterine rupture!" I say to Jane, "We have to go. I'm so sorry. I need to take you to the OR, and I need you to trust me. I think your uterus is ruptured." She is scared, eyes wide over the oxygen mask, but she nods.

How long can a baby live like this? How long do I have to get this baby out, undamaged? It depends on things I can't know right now: how much of the placenta remains attached to a normal uterine wall; how much blood the baby loses; how much blood the woman loses. It depends on location and luck. The answer to how much time I have is: go faster.

People rush to us, but we start to move without waiting for them. We leave her husband behind in the room; no time. As we roll, the charge nurse tells me that the OR is ready; the anesthesia resident is injecting medications down the syringe with one hand while pushing the bed with the other. We bang the doors to the OR open, and I hear "eight nine ten" as the tech finishes her instrument count. We roll Jane to the surgical bed in the usual chaos of people trying to help; we move her torso, then her legs. My OBGYN chief resident is already pouring surgical prep over her belly before Jane is settled on the surgical bed. The pediatric team is running in, getting quick details while they go to their corner and start to get ready. I get gloved and gowned while my chief resident throws a drape over Jane. That anesthesia bolus on the run is in, thank God, and Jane has adequate anesthesia before I have my gloves on.

Anesthesia tells me I'm safe to go, and then I go, knife on skin within 15 minutes of the baby's first fetal heart abnormality. Is it fast enough? Skin open, muscle open, some scar tissue, no time to stop; I see baby. No uterus as there should be; no thick muscular uterine wall, just baby floating in the belly, in a sea of blood. The baby is out, limp, blue; cord clamp placed; umbilical cord cut. Is that some movement as I hand her off? Please be some movement. I hand the baby off to the pediatricians. They take the baby off to the corner to start resuscitation. I hear them yell for more supplies; I hear them yell out some low numbers, bad numbers. Are they starting chest compressions?

Jane is bleeding, so we drag our attention back to her quickly. She's awake; she's been awake the whole time. I hear the anesthesia team murmuring to her softly. I say aloud that we have bleeding: "EBL [estimated blood loss] 1 liter already, not controlled." I lean over the patient and call out; I see Jane's brown eyes widen. I'm telling anesthesia we need a transfusion because I can't fix this quickly. I don't have time to explain to Jane, but I wasn't careful enough with my tone of voice and I'm sure she can hear the urgency. Anesthesia calls for help; they call for blood.

The chief resident and I pull at the uterus. Where is the top? Where is the bottom? What can we sew together? I find the ragged edges, finally, but we are having a hard time sewing much of it together; the scar ruptured in all directions, creating a stellate defect involving most of the front wall of the uterus. Will we have to do a hysterectomy? I know that's not what Jane wants, especially with this baby's fate still unknown. It's not what any of us want for her. But the bleeding doesn't stop; it's getting to the point of being dangerous for her. At some point, anesthesia gives Jane something to relax her, because when I lean over again, she is breathing on her own, but her eyes are closed and her face is relaxed. We've called up for 2 units of blood; no, make that 4.

Finally, we manage to find edges of tissue that are thick enough and piece the uterus together. The bleeding slows, and we add strength to the uterine wall we reconstituted out of frayed tissue, layer by layer.

In the middle of this, the baby is wheeled behind me so that Jane can see her. I note as the baby goes by that the baby is breathing on her own, that she didn't need to be intubated: that's good, that's hopeful. I keep sewing. The pediatricians stop by to briefly update

Jane and allow her a brief touch; Jane is awake enough to pass her hand into the incubator and pat the baby on the head; then the baby is rolled downstairs. I'm still sewing, and over an hour and 4 more units of blood later, we finish the surgery. Jane still has her uterus and has been stable the whole time; we roll her into the postanesthesia recovery unit (PACU) and go to find her family.

The next morning, before I go home, I stop by Jane's hospital room. I find out that the baby is being moved out of the neonatal intensive care unit (NICU) to the regular well-baby nursery today. It seems that we got there in time.

.   .   .

ON THE PHONE with my friend Sarah, I don't tell this story. To be truly statistically fair, I'd have to tell her 99 reassuring TOLAC stories for each upsetting rupture. But she needs to know what will be worrying her providers, so I ask her if she knows that she'll be trying a TOLAC, that she has options. I make sure she knows what a uterine rupture is and what the odds are. I do say something like "It doesn't happen often, but it also doesn't happen never. And when it happens, it can be very scary."

Sarah wants to be safe, but she also wants to avoid surgery. Given Sarah's first birth experience, I can understand wanting to wander into the forest. I can understand going one step beyond and rejecting all that Western medicine has to offer. Sometimes I fall into this trap myself.

.   .   .

BEVERLY HUGHES CAME to triage to be checked out for some high blood pressure values found in clinic. She was 37 weeks pregnant, her first baby. This was many years ago; I was a relatively new physician, determined not to repeat the mistakes of my elders. I wanted to avoid overmedicalization of birth; I wanted to leave people alone if they could be left alone.

Beverly looked okay, and her baby looked great. Her clinic blood pressure readings were high, that's true. But her blood pressure at our site was fine; her labs were normal, and she didn't feel unwell. On exam, Beverly's cervix was closed and firm, the cervix of a woman who would have a terrible 3-day induction of labor and end up with a cesarean delivery. I didn't want to do that, not unless I had a good reason.

And right that second—right that second—I didn't have a good reason. Beverly didn't meet criteria for preeclampsia. She had a couple of high blood pressure readings, sure, but nothing in my system; and they weren't 4 hours apart, as the definition of the diagnosis states. There was no protein in her urine and no signs of other organs under stress on her labs. It would have been reasonable to induce her for gestational hypertension, but recommendations at the time also allowed for continuing a pregnancy with gestational hypertension until almost 39 weeks; so it was also reasonable not to.[15] I didn't want that 3-day induction for her. I didn't want her to be at higher risk for that undesired cesarean after a failed induction. I didn't want her to use my name as a synonym for "shit" in three years.

I talked to Beverly, and together we made a plan. She could go home with a urine collection to check for protein. Absolutely, she could return in 2 days to drop it off and have her blood pressure checked. No, of course she wouldn't ignore a headache or decreased fetal movement.

That was the plan: she'd go home.

Two days later, I saw her name again while making my way to the inpatient ward. "Beverly Hughes: Eclampsia." She ended up coming into triage early, with a headache and without her urine test for protein, but the hospital didn't need it because she almost immediately had a grand mal seizure in triage. She skipped right over preeclampsia to the most severe form of the disease—eclampsia—which includes brain involvement.

The team stabilized her and took her right to the operating room because the fetal heart rate tracing looked distressed, even after the seizure ended. Beverly ended up with an emergent cesarean delivery and on magnesium. On the day I saw her name, she was in the post-anesthesia care unit. Her baby was in the NICU. Beverly was told that this was likely just a rough transition to ex utero life; she was told that permanent damage to the baby from the seizure, from the time she spent not breathing, was unlikely, but that we would only know for sure after time.

I spent a long time thinking about what if. What if I had recommended that Beverly be admitted and induced that night in triage? Perhaps she would have already delivered and never gotten sick. Even if she hadn't yet delivered, she would have at least been in the hospital. She would have been on magnesium to keep her from seizing. She would have gotten oxygen. She would have been with us.

Instead, I sent her home, a discharge order paved with the best intentions. Those 2 days that could have been spent getting her ready for a vaginal delivery were used up by the time she came back. I sent her away, and when she came back, she and her baby were just too sick.

I sent her away because I didn't want to do things to her. She ended up with all those things done to her. I tried to avoid this road, only to have her end up going down it at 100 miles per hour, the medical team chasing after her.

Maybe I could have given her a little bit of intervention and avoided a whole lot.

I hadn't done anything wrong; with another patient, I would have been right. Many times before and since, I have been right. I didn't do anything wrong, and yet I regret deeply what happened to her. And what is regret except for saying that you wouldn't do it that way, for this person, again?

.   .   .

I'M BACK ON the phone today with my friend Sarah, who makes me laugh. We talk about what she really wants; she doesn't really want a forest—too muddy. She doesn't even want a home birth. What she wants is a vaginal delivery; she wants it for this pregnancy, but also because she wants out of this whole surgical birth pathway. She wants to avoid surgery and scar tissue and placenta accreta.

But more than that, Sarah wants to feel secure and safe; and more than that, really, she wants to feel like she knows what's going on, that she's in charge, that it's her body, her labor, and her baby in a way that the first labor wasn't.

And Sarah is lucky: she lives in a suburb on the East Coast, in easy distance of more than one large medical center. She has options.

The thing is, I tell her, she needs a lot for a successful TOLAC. The TOLAC experience she's looking for requires a labor and delivery hospital that officially supports VBAC, which means they have the necessary resources, such as full-time anesthesia and all the resources required to provide an urgent cesarean. But that's only part of it: the medical context also needs to have a culture that supports VBAC. The safety net that makes that logistical and cultural support of VBAC possible is capability. The hospitals that are the best at VBAC are usually the ones that have everything they need to get a patient out of trouble if things go horribly wrong.

It feels like bad karma to think this way, like signing a prenup at the wedding: you don't want to think about the bad outcome, and you definitely don't want to think about uterine rupture during your VBAC. But let's think about this situation in a different way: if you're going on a trapeze, having a safety line means that you can let go; you can see what nature does; you can fly and come back to the ground when you want to.

That's what I mean, I tell Sarah. It's sort of counterintuitive, but it's just the way I see it happen a lot of the time. Particularly for the TOLAC experience—where you are trying to avoid the most invasive outcome—a large hospital, with beeping monitors and protocols, is sometimes the least interventionist because those hospitals have everyone and everything they need to take care of you quickly if things go wrong. And because they do, those big giant hospitals can relax and let things proceed in a way that smaller hospitals just can't. Because a big hospital manages TOLAC all the time, it has the resources to feel comfortable letting your body work.

Finally, I tell Sarah that if she has the patience to tolerate the setting and the right high-level hospital, I think that they can serve her well. If she can accept a little bit of intervention in the setting, she can avoid a lot.

. . .

How much of a large academic hospital can really be changed? The powerful large hospitals are hard to change because their very largeness and immobility is part of their power (see Chapter 9). They are vast machineries of administration and resources; 24-hour consultation but also protocols and beeping machines. Sarah asks me if there's any way to modify that giant hospital setting to make it more serviceable to her and her family. She realizes that she probably can't change the hospital itself, but she can change who she brings as her team.

Sarah and I start talking about a professional labor-support person, often known as a doula. The role of doula is as ancient as childbirth itself, but the modern equivalent dates to somewhere around the 1990s. In the setting of that exponentially increasing cesarean delivery rate, women started to hire other women to be their birth companions and advocate for them within a medical system that often felt that it didn't have their best interests at heart. It's an acknowledgment that the current medical providers—the doctors and nurses at the hospital—don't generally have the time or training for labor support and don't consider such work their responsibility. Thus, the modern role of doula was born: a woman who works professionally as a labor companion, offering emotional support, informational support, physical comfort measures, and advocacy throughout labor.[16]

Despite decades of development within the United States, the title of doula is not very standardized: many women have full certification; others are in training; and still others are not in pursuit of any formal training and are "lay" doulas. Similarly, there are a range of experiences I've had with doulas, almost all wonderful and one or two quite difficult. Most doulas take their advocacy work extremely seriously; most of the time, that's wonderful for the patient. Rarely, that advocacy work can get in the way of the medical care I'm trying to give. But some research also shows that doula care can decrease cesarean delivery and improve a wide array of maternal and newborn metrics. I've worked with many fabulous doulas who know that childbirth success can mean different things to different people and who can help a patient navigate the not-completely-low-risk situation of TOLAC.

When Sarah considers a return to the busy nurses and efficient epidurals, a land similar to that of her first birth, she is also considering utilizing a labor companion and advocate, someone who can help her labor at home while that's safe and who will help her and her husband translate their desires to the medical team. A regular doula may be your secret to success, I agree; but please try to make sure she's someone who's worked with TOLACs and who knows your definition of success: a repeat cesarean delivery is not to be avoided at all costs.

. . .

SARAH ENDS UP with a plan to get her care at the large hospital 10 miles away, where she also plans to be accompanied by her extremely dedicated, savvy, and down-to-earth doula. When I next talk to her, 36 weeks into her pregnancy, she sounds good.

"How do you feel?" I ask.

"I feel . . . I feel like I know what's going on this time," she says.

A month later, Sarah texts me a picture of a very new newborn with a gorgeous bald head and delicate curled hands. The picture is accompanied by a gleeful caption, all caps: LOOK WHAT I DID.

For the moment, I don't know how this baby was birthed, but I can feel the joy. That's all Sarah really wanted, and it's everything we all deserve.

7.

Stillbirth

When We Talk about Birth, We Need to Talk about Death

The unexpected stillbirth diagnosis happens most frequently in the triage area, the small emergency room that most hospitals run next to their labor and delivery units. Women come in with any number of complaints—weird mucus, a moment of lightheadedness, small amounts of bleeding, contractions. Some of these complaints are not terribly concerning; some of them may get an internal eye roll from the triage nurse because they're not even problems, much less emergencies.

Whatever brings a patient to the triage unit, she is always greeted by a triage nurse who screens her for urgency. One of the first questions the triage nurse asks is, "When did you last feel the baby move?" A number of women don't remember. It wasn't today. Maybe it was yesterday? Maybe the day before?

This is when the triage nurse steps away from the computer. Whatever the patient initially came for, the nurse now has something urgent on her mind. She grabs the doppler fetal heart rate monitor. She places it on the patient's belly. She doesn't get the fetal heart tones right away, so she starts moving the monitor around. Then maybe the nurse does hear something: boom–boom–boom. No, too slow; that's gotta be the maternal heartbeat. At this point, she is starting to worry. Does the patient sense that worry yet? The nurse starts asking the patient to turn to one side; at the same time, the nurse calls out for the doctor to come and bring the ultrasound machine: "I need help finding a fetal heart." Sometimes, after she turns the patient and repositions the monitor, the triage nurse hears the heart: boom–boom, boom–boom, quick and in the 130s and different enough from the woman's for us to know that we have the right one.

But sometimes, even with movement and repositioning, the nurse hasn't found the fetal heartbeat. The nurse asks the patient to move quickly to a triage bed. Quickly, she now talks with the urgency we feel in this kind of situation: a sticky, dishonest urgency. There likely isn't any reason to hurry. Either it's a mistake—technical issues prevented our hearing the heartbeat, but everything is fine—or it's not a mistake, it's real, and it's already too late.

But the nurse doesn't move slowly and calmly because each moment that we don't know—is the pregnancy still alive?—is unbearable. The tension between "Everything is fine" and "Nothing will ever be fine again" must be resolved; it's impossible to live there, in the space where we don't know, for very long. And lurking behind the urgency, the doubt: what if, what if this is the minute when it's not too late?

The nurse walks with the patient to the closest empty bed. The patient feels the worry now; she hears the urgency. The nurse tries listening again while she waits for the intern to roll over the gigantic ultrasound machine and get it to boot up.

Once the machine is on, the intern stands with the ultrasound probe. She has been working in triage for three months; she is the second stop for most patients, after the triage nurse. She has gotten much better at certain things, but she knows she is still new. The intern also feels the worry, transmitted to her through the nurse's tone of voice, her quick movements. Maybe this is the first time this new doctor has been in this situation. She is scared of what she will see and of what she won't. She is most scared that she won't know what she is seeing.

The intern puts the ultrasound probe on the patient's belly. Sometimes she finds the fetal heart, moving quickly. There it is. Baby has its spine up, and that plus an anterior placenta and maternal obesity made the heartbeat hard to find. That's all it was. There it is. The intern, the nurse, and the patient all take some breaths and make some small talk, chatting away their unspoken relief.

But sometimes the intern puts the ultrasound probe on and she can't find that flutter of the heart. She tries not to panic; she remembers what she's been taught and tries to find the fetal head, and then the spine, and follows it to the ribs. There's the fetal stomach; the heartbeat should really be right here. It really should. She looks and looks. And only when she realizes how hard she's looking for something that is always—always—so obvious, that's when she realizes she's looking for something that isn't there anymore.

In many hospitals, the protocol for diagnosing a stillbirth requires that an attending make the diagnosis: not a resident, not a nurse. This time, it happens that I am chatting on the labor floor when the intern comes running to find me. She needs me, she needs me *now*. There's that urgency again; it's not a clinical urgency; it is too late, it was already too late hours ago. It's the urgency of truth, of ending the uncertainty that the patient is living with in this moment; the urgency of beginning the grief.

The intern pours the story out to me and ends with the thought that maybe she's just wrong? Maybe she's just so poor at ultrasound? She wants so badly to be wrong; she prefers for it to be her fault if that means that something here would be salvageable, if we could make this not be true.

I don't think the intern is wrong. I think she knows what she saw. And though I know it's too late, I feel that same urgency, too. I walk quickly, half running, fueled by dread.

I draw back the curtain in triage. I introduce myself. I sit down by the side of the patient. I put the probe on her belly. I look around, though I see within 10 seconds what I am looking for. I am thorough, though I already know. By my inaction, the nurse and intern know, too. By now, the patient knows, too: something is very wrong.

I take a deep breath. I say, "I have some terrible news for you. There is no heartbeat. The baby is dead. The baby died." I try to speak clearly. I try to convey the irreversibility of what has happened. There should be clarity; it is the very least I can do.

Often, the keening starts while I'm still talking, a high sound behind my words. Sometimes it's sobbing. Sometimes it's screaming. Sometimes the patient screams at me; sometimes the patient's father or husband or mother screams at me or the nurse or the heavens. Sometimes they beseech me, the ultrasound machine, the heavens for something different. Find the heartbeat, they sometimes say. Wake the baby up. Try again.

If they ask, I show them the ultrasound, the black cloverleaf of stillness in the chest in place of the constant movement of a beating heart. I say the same thing, that the baby is dead, in different ways, again and again. If they desire, I leave and come back and say it again.

Eventually, they are ready to ask more questions: Why? How? What comes next? The only one I can usually answer at this point is the last one. I tell them we recommend admission and workup to try to figure out what happened and to make sure that nothing danger-ous to the patient herself is going on. And despite everything, we still need to get the baby out. We recommend induction of labor, if they will allow it, as soon as possible. Eventually, they are ready to accept the move to our labor floor, to an IV placement, to lab work. They head to labor room 3 for the rest of the worst day of their life.

.   .   .

LIKE ANY DEATH, stillbirth is the end result of a million different possibilities of what might have gone wrong. Some stillbirths are long foretold: an abnormal brain or an abnormal heart detected on an early ultrasound. Sometimes we already have chromosomal results on a pregnancy; we see the devastating genetic loss or gain, and we already know exactly what to expect. Those stillbirths are a large percentage of the losses that we diagnose. But others are unexpected: a normal preg-nancy, moving along without complications, until one day it doesn't; a fetus that is perfect—was perfect—except that it's dead.

In medical terms, stillbirth is called intrauterine fetal demise (IUFD). It's how we describe a pregnancy that is lost late in gesta-tion, usually after 20 weeks of pregnancy. Stillbirth is not preterm labor or any of the other ways that pregnancies can go wrong where we end up with a dead baby after delivery. It is, instead, when somehow, at some time, the fetal heart just stops beating. This happens once every 170 to 200 births,[1] which is to say it hasn't happened to everyone you know, but it's probably happened to someone you know or to someone who someone you know knows. I've diagnosed and delivered too many stillbirths to count. Too many.

Whatever the cause of the stillbirth, making the diagnosis and telling the patient is just the beginning. Here is the thing that medical providers learn very early in their work: the worst day of a patient's life can always, always get worse.

The baby is dead, but why? Perhaps the patient has an infection inside her uterus; the infection killed the baby and is on the way to making the patient herself septic. Perhaps the placenta started to separate, a placental abruption, with bleeding between the placenta and the uterine wall it was attached to. Once the placenta separates too much, the fetus dies from lack of oxygen; but if the bleeding continues, the woman herself will be in danger. Or perhaps the patient has uncontrolled, severe preeclampsia; the loss of the fetus was just the harbinger of the elevated blood pressure, seizures, and strokes that are starting to develop within her body. Perhaps it's none of these— just terrible luck, just a bad placenta, nothing else. But we can't know until we determine whether this was the end or just the sentinel event. Sometimes something more ominous is on the way. Sometimes, this is not the end of the worst day of her life but just the start.

What needs to be orchestrated now isn't simple. We still need to get the baby out. We need to guide a woman who may be getting very sick through a safe labor and a safe delivery. Complications need to be avoided: bleeding, infection, need for a hysterectomy that would mean no pregnancies ever again.

It can feel barbaric to ask a woman to go through this; I've been asked whether a patient can go to sleep, have a cesarean, and wake up with the whole experience behind her. The answer is it's feasible but unwise; that wouldn't be the safest way out. Going to sleep with general anesthesia is still one of the most dangerous things a pregnant woman can do. Major surgery is still major surgery and has risks, including risks for later reproductive life (see Chapter 6). What generally needs to happen, then, is labor and delivery. We can try to make it as painless or even as muzzy as possible with medications and epidurals, but we can't make it unnecessary.

On the day of a stillbirth and the subsequent labor and delivery, I feel like hooded Charon, a guide across the river of death. This woman needs to be steered through this birth that is already a death; she needs to land safely on the other side. The medical team needs to guide a patient across that river, through death and back to life. But we are hooded, anonymous, invisible. The patient usually does not want—cannot deal with—the knowledge of what else is going wrong or can go wrong. She doesn't really want to know me or who I am or that I am. The patient doesn't see the riverman as we help her cross this dark river; she can't see the perils in the water; it is not the time to ask her to recognize our efforts.

We row across, slowly, painstakingly, and deposit her on the other side safely. She will never be grateful for this trip; it is still the worst day of her life. But having it only be the worst day of her life is the sole gift that Charon can give; and sometimes it takes everything we have to give it.

Most of the time, women with a stillbirth are admitted to labor room 3. There is a sign posted on their door so that all the staff is reminded of the sadness in this room; we don't waltz in chatting or try to strap on a fetal heart monitor. The patient gets some oxytocin and then an epidural. She is awake when she delivers her baby because this is the safest way. She has to push, though usually not for too long, because these dead babies are often early or small. After delivery, in that quiet room with no cry, we wrap the baby up after it's born, as we would a live baby; we put a striped hat on its head. We make a small neat package of it; it can look like a live baby, sometimes, from across the room.

After the birth, the patient doesn't have to see the baby, but she can. Studies have shown that patients who don't physically say goodbye sometimes regret it later; sometimes they are angry that they didn't take this opportunity.[2] The staff takes pictures of the baby for her, work that is both gruesome and important. We make her a keepsake box, which some patients never open and some view as their most precious possession. Sometimes, we ask whether she wants an amniocentesis before delivery; we can get cells, uncontaminated by birth, to try to give us a diagnosis. Even harder, even more macabre, we ask whether she wants an autopsy of the baby's body. Often, this can give us the best shot at knowing what happened and why and preventing it at future pregnancies. In my experience, almost nobody says yes to the autopsy.

We have to discuss a million more things: Does she want genetic tests sent? Does she want to bury the baby's body? Will there be a funeral? A cremation? Leave the small body in the hospital morgue for disposal? All of these details need to be discussed and forms filled out, signed, stamped.

After all this, the patient is usually moved to a private room on the gynecology floor, far from the postpartum unit where all the healthy babies are. After 1 or 2 days, she is discharged home, usually with an appointment for therapy or for a grieving support group.

That's what usually happens, when everything goes as well as it can, when Charon successfully navigates the river. But sometimes our patient is already pulled into the water after her baby, submerged in the river of death, halfway and sometimes all the way in.

.   .   .

IT WAS 2 P.M. on a Friday afternoon. Valerie Prava had come in at 10 a.m. with abdominal pain that had started only 15 minutes earlier; she had called 911 and been brought to our hospital as fast as possible. In her first pregnancy, now 40 weeks and a few days pregnant, Valerie was grunting in pain that didn't come and go like contractions, but was constant, without relief. Valerie came alone.

When we put the ultrasound on Valerie's belly, we saw right away that there was no heartbeat for the fetus. We also saw a giant blood collection behind the placenta, pushing the placenta off. Valerie had what was called a concealed abruption. In her case, it was so large that the placenta was no longer attached; without a placenta, the fetus had no oxygen and had quickly died. The abruption was concealed in that Valerie had no external bleeding; the massive collection of blood was contained within her uterus. All Valerie had was tremendous pain as her uterus stretched and reacted to the blood collecting inside it.

We told Valerie about the baby's death; but we were already moving fast. Valerie's vital signs were already showing signs of blood loss. Her heart was beating fast, and her blood pressure was a little bit low; this is how a patient looks when her body is starting to have difficulty compensating for the lack of blood within the blood vessels, when she is about to crash. Valerie was crying from pain, and she began crying in grief and fear as well. She wept and begged for pain medicine, all at the same time. We started an IV. We gave her some morphine. We sent her blood to the lab, stat; we sent a doctor down to the lab to tell them that we needed those results immediately.

The labs results showed that Valerie's hemoglobin was low, and her clotting tests showed that her blood was on the verge of no lon- ger clotting well: too many of her body's clotting factors were already being used up trying to stop the bleeding in her uterus. Without clotting factors, the bleeding in the uterus would only get worse.

The team started to transfuse Valerie with blood but also with blood products that included clotting factors. Valerie needed to deliver quickly: she wouldn't stop bleeding into her uterus until it was empty. The team huddled around the nursing station: obstet- rics, maternal-fetal medicine, anesthesia, nursing.

They could take her to the operating room, which would be the quickest delivery. They could perform a cesarean delivery. But taking an unstable patient to the operating room is usually a bad idea; add- ing stress to her already stressed body can push her over the edge.

Should they try to get her to a vaginal delivery? Often preg- nancies affected by abruption deliver very quickly; blood generally irritates the uterus and causes contractions. The team decided to transfuse her aggressively and start oxytocin; they would give it 2 hours. If she wasn't well on the way to delivering by then, they would head to the operating room.

Oxytocin and transfusions were started. Valerie's cervix was closed, then 1 centimeter dilated; as she dilated, she began to bleed vaginally. But it wasn't enough: her uterus was also rising in her belly, filling with more and more blood. Before the 2 hours were up, the team was having trouble keeping up with her blood loss. They were running out of time. The team decided to head to the operating room.

In the operating room, Valerie wasn't stable enough to get an

epidural. General anesthesia is not the safest option for most pregnant women, but for Valerie, we had no safer option. Valerie went all
the way to sleep and had a tube placed down her throat. The team
positioned her on the table and started a quick cesarean delivery.
The operating room was tense and quiet without pediatricians or
family members; just murmured communication between the two
obstetric surgeons and updates from the anesthesiologist about Valerie's vital signs.

One minute after skin incision, the uterus was opened. Three
liters of clot and blood were removed, and a fetus, and a placenta. The
uterus was a strange purplish color, not its usual beefy red, probably
from having so much blood forced into its muscular wall. The muscle
of the uterine wall was also not working well; it was boggy and floppy.
Even after being emptied, the uterus wouldn't contract. And so Valerie
continued bleeding. She bled; the rate of transfusion was increased.
All the medicines useful to help a uterus clamp down were given, and
then given again. There was some improvement but not enough.

Now 10 minutes had passed since the uterus was emptied; now
15 minutes. Surgical techniques were initiated at the same time: a
large balloon was placed in the uterus to try to provide pressure
from within. Valerie continued to bleed.

The surgical team knew that continuing to try to save Valerie's
uterus might be futile; and worse, it might cost the time needed to
save her life. As a last-ditch effort, they decided to try a B-Lynch
compression suture. If that didn't work, they would proceed with a
hysterectomy. Valerie continued to bleed.

The team didn't talk about what this meant—that Valerie would
wake up with no baby and no uterus. At this point, they were just
trying to get to the part where she could wake up.

The team called for a hysterectomy tray, for all the instruments they would need to take out the bleeding uterus. They called for the large hysterectomy retractor to better visualize the deep areas of the pelvis while performing a hysterectomy. With those on the way, the team then quickly sewed a B-Lynch suture, stitching around the bottom of the uterus like a belt, and then two large sutures over the shoulders of the enormous bluish uterus. The B-Lynch compressed the uterus down around the intrauterine balloon in all directions.

The bleeding slowed. Did it slow enough? For the first time in half an hour, everyone stopped. They watched. They watched some more. After a few minutes, the surgical team agreed that it was slow enough, good enough, for now. No hysterectomy, for now. The team quickly closed Valerie's abdomen, leaving a drain in to empty any further blood that might collect. Valerie had, by this point, received somewhere around 10 units of blood, enough to have replaced her own blood volume twice over.

Valerie was taken to the ICU. She was kept asleep through the next 48 hours, a roller coaster of replacing more blood products and adjusting medications to deal with the enormous shock her body had suffered. The obstetrics team checked on her every hour, then every 2 hours: her vaginal bleeding was moderate, then light. The abdominal drain showed blood, then watery fluid; eventually, it drained nothing.

After a day, we deflated the intrauterine balloon in stages, removing 100 milliliters of fluid at a time, to allow the uterus to contract around it; eventually, it was removed. Valerie's bleeding remained light.

Valerie spiked a fever. Her white blood count was abnormal, incredibly high, either a result of the stress her body had gone through or the result of a serious infection. She was transferred to the CT unit and then back; no huge infection was seen. We increased her antibiotic coverage from three medications to four.

That night, Valerie's heart rate started to normalize. She received 2 or 3 more units of blood, but for the first time, her blood count went up as it should. We had caught up.

Two days after her surgery, the ICU team woke Valerie up. They removed her breathing tube. Valerie was breathing well; she was alert and talking, though her voice was scratchy from having a tube between her vocal cords for 48 hours. Valerie remembered almost everything about that afternoon 2 days ago; for her it was 5 minutes ago but also a million years ago. Valerie remembered the pain and that the baby was dead. She was told what had happened in the time since: that she almost died, too, more than once. She was told that she still had her uterus; that we worked hard to save it. She said, hoarsely, that she understood. After a pause, she said that she would be grateful to the team another day; she just couldn't be happy about it, not right now.

· · ·

AT DIAGNOSIS OF a stillbirth, there are two questions that we can almost never answer: Why? How? What we're all really asking is, could this stillbirth have been prevented?

Sometimes the answer is no. There was a problem with the fetus, a problem like an extra chromosome 18 or a series of small deletions in the base pairs that make up an important gene or a complicated series of heart malformations. There was never any way to save that pregnancy.

But much of the time, the answer is maybe.

The medical world has been trying for years to figure out how stillbirths happen and why. There is a long list of maternal risk factors that increase the risk of stillbirth, including weight, cigarette smoking, advanced maternal age, multiple gestation, medical complications such as hypertension and diabetes, and, most horrifyingly, racial ethnicity (see Chapter 10 for a longer discussion of how this is true, and why).

Many stillbirths have almost nothing to do with the fetus. The fetus in those pregnancies is in perfect working order. The problem in those pregnancies is with what supports the fetus, the combination of maternal and placental blood supply that we call the uteroplacental unit. For life before delivery, the uteroplacental unit is the only source for the fetus's food, drink, and, crucially, oxygen. If blood isn't getting to the uterus or from the uterus into the placenta, then the fetus can't get what it needs to live.

The uteroplacental unit can be affected by anything that affects blood supply throughout the mother's body. Diseases such as long-standing hypertension or diabetes will mean that the maternal blood vessels that grow to meet the placenta are not wide enough.

Sometimes the placenta itself isn't working well, perhaps because the placenta has a genetic problem that the fetus doesn't share or because the placenta is the first example of planned obsolescence: humans make this miraculous little organ, but we make it to last only 40 or so weeks. At some point after 42 weeks or so, the placenta starts to fill with calcium and the vessels become stiff, and the whole thing stops working quite so well.[3]

It's important to understand the uteroplacental unit because if the uteroplacental unit is the problem, then modern medicine has a solution: delivery. If we know that this fetus is in trouble, we can deliver the baby, instantly rendering the placenta moot. The baby may be early; the baby may have problems because of that; but delivery will mean that the baby will no longer need the placenta and no longer be dependent on the uterus. Deciding when the myriad risks of preterm birth are more dangerous than the one big risk of a pregnancy suffering from uteroplacental insufficiency is one of the thorniest problems in maternal-fetal medicine.

What all this means is that many of those stillbirths attributable to uteroplacental insufficiency are, we think, preventable. The baby, if we had known, if we had gotten her out, would have lived. Emotionally speaking, a preventable tragedy arguably feels more tragic than an unpreventable one. For those physicians whose job it is to not allow these things to happen, it feels like the ultimate dereliction of duty. It is the very thing we have trained for years and provided care for months to avoid. And this feeling of horror and guilt isn't specific to a particular patient; I feel it when I'm taking care of a patient with an IUFD who wasn't under my care during her pregnancy or even one whose loss was years ago. As a profession, as a discipline, we failed her.

In this way, the doctor taking care of a patient with an IUFD is also experiencing a tragedy, a loss of faith. It's from a different perspective: from the outside; it is of a much lesser degree, and we all know that. It's not my baby, and it's not my body. It's not, in the end, my life. But it is, nonetheless, a grief that we are adjacent to.

For providers, it is a grief we are next to not just once, but again and again. It is a strange and repeated sorrow. We deliver a silent baby; we wrap up a small, neat, dead package. Again and again—sometimes once a month, sometimes once every six months—we come to work, pull that hood over our head, and prepare to steer someone new across the river of death. And over time, it can become harder and harder to come to the riverside, oar in hand.

· · ·

Today is different.

Today, as I usually do before coming to the hospital on the weekend at the luxurious hour of 8:00 a.m., I sit in my pajamas with my hot cocoa and log on to the computer to see who is on the labor floor, to see what kind of day I have in store. But today, when I check, I see that in room 1 there is a woman, Clara Gimondi. She is there with a 32-week IUFD, admitted by the overnight doctor, Dr. Howard.

Clara was two months before her due date. She came in for a routine visit, without complaints, and there were no fetal sounds on the monitor, and then there was a still fetal heart, that nonmoving cloverleaf shape, on ultrasound. She is now there to have her labor induced. No preeclampsia, no bleeding; no obvious reason for now.

Sitting at home with my hot cocoa, I sit back, frozen in my chair, paralyzed by how much I don't want to go to work. It's not that it's hard to take care of these women: it is, but I've prided myself on being really good at it. It's not just that I can be kind or patient, though those skills are important. It's more that I know that I'm not terribly important in that room; I'm a bit player in this large tragedy. I know how to go about my work of keeping a patient safe, of being available, but fading into the background. This is something I'm proud of, because it is an awful and difficult thing to be able to do.

But today is different for me, because I am 11 weeks pregnant with my first pregnancy. Things have been hard for me—infertility, emergent surgery, complications—and yet, so far, to my eternal surprise, I have not miscarried or bled to death or somehow managed to mess this up. Every chance I get, I check my stomach with the ultrasound; I am always surprised to see the small flicker of that living pregnancy.

As I brush my teeth in the early-morning dimness, I am reeling with how badly I want to stay out of this woman's room. For my own pregnancy, I have worried about miscarriage, preterm labor, preeclampsia, delivering a previable infant, and genetic problems— all the things that OBGYNs are both privileged and doomed to see. And the worrying thus far has been protective, you see, because I'm doing okay so far.

But I forgot to worry about the pregnancy dying inside of me at 32 weeks, so Clara's diagnosis catches me like a well-thrown punch. I know that IUFDs are not contagious; I know that. And yet. I am desperate to stay out of her room. I don't want to have to look into her eyes, I don't want to share her pain the way I usually do. In the end, I just want my happy pregnancy, my eventual healthy baby, and I don't want to look at the other side.

As I put on scrubs and clip my pager to my belt and snap my ID onto my collar, I work myself out of it. You're being irrational, I tell myself, and unfair. She deserves better; she deserves everything you have to give her. It will be easier, I tell myself, because no one knows that you're pregnant yet. I work myself toward her, away from self-ishness back to compassion.

When I finally walk through the doors of labor and delivery, Dr. Howard meets me at the nursing desk. "She delivered overnight; it was really fast, and really uncomplicated, it happened at 4 a.m. I don't think you're going to need to see her. She's going to go to the GYN floor now; she wants to go home tomorrow, so I'm getting her paperwork done."

"Oh," I say. "Well, that's something, that's good, I guess. Do you need me to do anything?"

Doctor Howard says no, it's all done, and goes home to sleep, maybe to have a couple of glasses of wine.

Half an hour later, the nurse comes to get me. There's one last form to fill out; Dr. Howard must have left it in the room. It needs to be signed by a physician. It's the disposition of remains, the form where the family decides whether they want the baby's body for a funeral or service or whether they want the hospital to take care of it.

This is a big decision and one that families often regret. At the time of delivery, they often sign over the body; they just want to be done, just get out with their hands empty. But later, they can be furious, made inconsolable by their empty hands; later, they may regret that they had no ceremony to remember, no gravesite to visit.

The nurse tells me that Clara has decided. Social work has spent a lot of time with the patient and her husband. They just need a physician to witness the document.

"All right," I say. I falter; I'd rather not. But I stand up. I go into room 1. I say hello. I say, "I'm sorry for your loss." Clara is dressed in sweatpants and a striped heavy sweater, not in a hospital gown, her hands balled up inside her sleeves. Her hair is in a loose ponytail. Her husband sits next to her, hands loose in his lap, his face pale. Clara has the form in front of her.

I say, "Do you have any questions about this form?" Clara says no. She has checked off option A; the hospital will dispose of her baby's remains.

I could ask her if she's sure.

I could say: Some people regret it later.

I could say: Call us if you change your mind.

But I don't. I say, "I'm here all day and all night. Please let us know if there is anything we can do to help."

She looks up at me as she passes the paper back. Her hand does not touch mine. "There is nothing," she says. I nod.

She and her husband, composed, fully dressed, are sitting next to each other on the bed, not touching. Nobody looking at them would know what they went through last night, what they are going through today and tomorrow and for the rest of their lives. I walk to the door and walk out.

I put a hand to my stomach after the door closes behind me. I feel dirty and undeserving and sad. When I go to the bathroom, I am surprised to find that I am not bleeding. Today, I do not go to listen to my pregnancy with the ultrasound; the luck that I have had is enough.

. . .

THIS GRIEF THAT obstetric caregivers experience with each stillbirth is peripheral but individual. We are never the center of any of these tragedies, but each provider experiences it differently with each patient, each time. But the effect is also collective, which means that, as a discipline, modern obstetrics is often guided by the avoidance of stillbirth, by the instinct to keep this tragedy away from our patients and perhaps also from ourselves. Such is the power of stillbirth. And such is its power that even the mention of it is traumatic. It is rare for us to overtly mention this possibility when we see patients; we don't explain exactly why we're recommending a certain course of action, exactly what it is that we're worried could happen.

Stillbirth has thus become the unspoken shadow behind many of our most technical and coldly written protocols. Once you know this, you see how almost every pregnancy is touched by the fear of stillbirth, how much of the obstetric care we give is secretly, silently, constantly aimed at preventing this problem.

For example, the risk of stillbirth is a large part of why something as common as postdate fetal monitoring exists. We recommend that patients come in for fetal monitoring after 40 weeks because the risk of stillbirth goes up a little. Patients are offered inductions of labor after 41 to 42 weeks because after that point the risk of stillbirth goes up a lot.[4] The risk of stillbirth is why women with diabetes or hypertension—with their higher risk of a compromised uteroplacental unit—spend so much time in fetal monitoring; it's why those patients will have induction recommended for them well before their due date. The risk of stillbirth is the unspoken reason behind a million different decisions made regarding both low-risk and high-risk pregnancies.

In many low-income countries, about half of stillbirths occur during labor and delivery, largely because of a lack of skilled birthing attendants or capability for urgent cesarean delivery. However, in high-income countries, where monitoring in labor is the norm[5] and cesarean deliveries are generally available in most hospitals providing obstetric care (in most hospitals, but not enough; see Chapter 6), the discussion has shifted to other causes.

In places such as the United States, nowhere is the risk of stillbirth less talked about yet more significant than in the problem of fetus with intrauterine growth restriction (IUGR). IUGR technically refers to fetuses under the 10th percentile. But of course, 10 percent of normal babies will be under the 10th percentile; that's how statistics works. Most of those babies are doing fine; that size is their genetic destiny. Those babies are called "constitutionally small"; for those babies, small is just how they are supposed to be.

But some of those small fetuses are not supposed to be small. They're under the 10th percentile because they are not getting quite enough calories. Their uteroplacental unit is not working well for them as a food delivery system. There are a whole bunch of ways that we try to distinguish the constitutionally small fetus from those that are really, truly not getting enough to eat: using complicated Doppler flow calculations of the vessels of the umbilical cord; assessing measurements of brain blood flow via ultrasound measurements; watching how the growth of the belly compares with the growth of the brain. None of these tools are perfect; all of them can fail us.

So we have to continue to pay attention. Those fetuses that are small because they are not getting enough calories are also at risk for further deterioration of uteroplacental function. They may start getting less fluid through the umbilical cord. In that case, we start to see oligohydramnios, or low amniotic fluid volume around the baby. Amniotic fluid in third trimester is just fetal urine (sterile, clean fetal urine), so when fetuses don't get enough hydration through the umbilical cord, they don't pee. In many ways, oligohydramnios is analogous to having a dry diaper in a newborn: it signals that the baby is dehydrated and that we should worry.

The last function of the placenta, after calories and fluid, is oxygen: bringing oxygen from the maternal blood and ventilating the carbon dioxide that the fetus manufactures. Fetuses can live for weeks with low calories and for days (or even weeks) with low fluid; but oxygen is something fetuses need every minute. When the oxygen is lost, that is when we can end up with a stillbirth.

Thus, once IUGR is diagnosed, and especially if it's accompanied by oligohydramnios, the protocols are to watch these small fetuses like a hawk. We sometimes bring them in once a week, or twice a week, for fetal monitoring and ultrasound. Sometimes, in cases of very early and very extreme growth restriction, we admit the pregnant woman into the hospital, because now we need to monitor twice or sometimes three times a day. If the pregnancy is at term or close to term, we recommend induction or even sometimes a cesarean delivery. We will often even deliver early, weighing the risks of prematurity against the risks of IUFD and choosing the risks of prematurity, though they may be terrible. Such is the catastrophe of IUFD: it is worth doing anything to avoid it.

Our tools are imperfect, and medical providers know that. Ultrasound measurements have an error rate of 10 to 15 percent, even in the best of hands, which means that some IUGR fetuses that we follow and sweat over and hospitalize are born at a normal weight. Many of them are little but healthy, just constitutionally small; we know that, too. We just can't tell with certainty who will be who. That's the recipe for anxiety, I think: the worry caused by a legitimate possibility, minus the ability to completely reassure anyone that it won't happen. And because we can't know for sure, for an obstetric provider, the risk of stillbirth hovers over all of these pregnancies.

But even in these pregnancies of IUGR, even when we are overtly watching the fetus for signs that it might be getting ready to die, we say things like "I'm concerned about the fetal growth." We almost never say something like "Your fetus is measuring less than the tenth percentile, which means that you have approximately double the risk of the baby dying inside your uterus." Stillbirth is so catastrophic that even the mention of it—the sheer reminder that it is real and possible—is traumatic for everyone in the room. Instead, we talk about birth; and when we talk about birth, we rarely mention death.

In this way, we ask women to bear the cost of this anxiety over stillbirth—both theirs and ours—while rarely fully explaining why. And the cost of this collective anxiety is high. It's a woman who loses her job because she has to come twice a week for an hour of monitoring. It's a cesarean delivery performed for a failed induction at 37 weeks, and a wound infection from that cesarean delivery. It's a 37-week baby admitted to the NICU with breathing problems after an induction for IUGR—breathing problems that she wouldn't have had if born 2 weeks later.

We do not talk of death during those prenatal visits, ultrasound appointments, and inductions of labor. The high cost can seem egregious. "Why am I coming in for monitoring?" my patients grumble. "Everything is always fine." She's not wrong; today everything is fine. Everything may always be fine, and often would have been fine, even without any of our costly interventions. But the unspoken consequence on the other side of that tally is stillbirth, so weighty that it pulls almost every equation down as soon as it is considered, even when it goes unmentioned. Any equation that includes stillbirth will lean heavily toward obstetric intervention.

Is all this anxiety and care and monitoring working? In some ways, yes—or at least, probably. Around the world, the overall stillbirth rate is going down.[6] Most of this improvement is attributable to provision of basic prenatal and labor and delivery care. We do see improvement with our monitoring and early delivery of patients with diabetes and hypertensive diseases.

But in some important ways, the anxiety and care are not working. When we focus on the particulars of intrauterine growth restriction, the improvement in stillbirth rate is not as clear. Overall, intervention near term may be helpful. However, multiple studies have shown that immediate intervention in growth-restricted fetuses did not meaningfully change outcomes over waiting longer to deliver; outcomes that remained the same included death.[7] In these studies, delivery just meant that a stillbirth was exchanged for a neonatal demise: death, either way. More studies are being done every day to better understand how we can intervene in ways that will help and not hurt. We are not there yet, however much we want to be.

In the end, I also have the evidence of my own experience and of Clara's and of Valerie's. It is as medically true as anything else that Clara's baby might have had a chance if we had known at 28 weeks that it was struggling, if we had been following closely, if we had delivered. It is true, also, that Valerie's baby would be alive if she had been born a week earlier and that Valerie would not have gone through surgery and an ICU stay and almost died.

This is what we hold in our hands with stillbirth: our fear and our power, but also ultimately our powerlessness. Remember that urgency, the sweaty dishonest urgency I felt when I was too late, too powerless to change anything; that need to look, to name the grief anyway? For obstetric providers, that murmur of urgency exists every day, everywhere, for better or for worse. The fear of stillbirth pushes us to act, urges us to do better, pulls us to find ways to prevent this outcome; at the same time, we almost never mention it by name. It is silent but never absent.

All of us within this work of obstetrics have been Charon, often many times, always too many times. We have all rowed patients across the river of death, through a birth that is already death, to the other side. We know this is holy, necessary work. If we need to, we can do it again tomorrow and the next day and the next; we have, and we will. But what we really want is never to do it again. We want to walk, with our patients, away from the river of death, back to life.

GOING INTO THE HOSPITAL (OR STAYING OUT)

8.

Informed Consent

Sign Here and Don't Ask Too Many Questions

I know a woman who is extremely competent, has a PhD, and is the boss of an office full of people. She always knows what to do next and how she's going to do it and has a 14-step itemized plan to make it happen.

Last year, after 2 days of labor, at 8 centimeters dilated, at 4 a.m., she signed a paper agreeing to a cesarean delivery. She remembers that a doctor talked to her, or at her, right before she signed, but she can tell you nothing of what that doctor said. She—a woman who has never ever skipped a footnote in any book she's ever read—did not read the paper handed to her. She scribbled her signature at the bottom of the form balanced on the back of a tissue box while an IV pulled at her elbow. This woman has no idea what she signed or why, exactly at that moment, her labor needed to be over; she doesn't know why she wasn't offered a cesarean earlier, or later, or never.

She's not upset about the cesarean delivery; she thinks she

needed it, and she and her baby are healthy. She just finds the whole experience . . . weird. Disempowering. So removed from her normal life. "What exactly was that?" she asked.

"That was informed consent," I told her. "It says that you were informed about the procedure and that you consented."

"Neither of those words is being used in any way that I understand them," she replied.

. . .

WE LIVE IN a world where we click "agree" to the terms of the website without reading them; we sign pieces of paper giving up essential rights before we go skiing or bungee jumping; we dismiss the flight attendants' safety check because "they just have to tell us about that." In medicine, too, I stand in front of a patient with a piece of paper reviewing the risks, benefits, and alternatives to surgery. I am asking the patient, in a moment of her greatest vulnerability, to indicate that she knows that this could be the right decision or a devastatingly wrong one.

Why do we perform this ritual of informed consent? Doctors do this because we have to, for legal protection and to protect ourselves and our hospitals, but that's only part of the reason. Doctors ask for consent because modern society believes in patient autonomy: that people receiving medical care should choose what happens—and what doesn't happen—to their bodies. But medical informed consent is very easy to do wrong and almost impossible to do right.

One of the ways consent goes awry is that adjective "informed." That adjective is there because genuine consent, the way people generally understand it, requires access to information. That information needs to be unbiased, free of coercion, and, most importantly, true. For most of medical history, informed consent suffered from a lack of information: patients were told little about their procedure, about the risks, about the alternatives. Inadequate information essentially led to inadequate consent.

This still happens today, but usually not for malevolent or careless reasons. In a true emergency, for example, where a minute or two might make a difference to a person's life, informed consent is a challenge.

Consider the case of operative vaginal delivery. Approximately 3.3 percent of deliveries in the United States are operative vaginal deliveries.[1] That category of delivery includes forceps deliveries and vacuum deliveries—basically, any time a delivery is vaginal but doesn't occur under the power of the maternal push alone. Of those operative vaginal deliveries, the reason for the intervention is often a nonreassuring fetal heart tracing—a fetus so stressed by the last stages of labor that there's real concern for insufficient oxygen. What should informed consent look like in that situation?

. . .

ONE WINTRY NIGHT, I was on call. My only patient needed a cesarean delivery, which I finished up at around 11 p.m. As I came out of the operating room, the midwife on call, Helen, was waiting for me. Helen is a very experienced midwife, so the list of reasons she would be looking for me was a very short one: either she had a patient who needed a cesarean delivery or one who needed an operative vaginal delivery.

"I have a patient who came in just 2 hours ago, first baby; she's in room 4. She's fully dilated. She's pushing, and pushing well," Helen says, "but I don't love the tracing. Every time she pushes, the baby has a dip in the heart rate. It was worrisome enough that I had her stop pushing until you got out of the OR. The tracing is a little better while we're waiting, but I think she needs to have this baby faster. I want you to come in and consider whether you would offer a forceps or vacuum."

"What's the station?" I ask. Operative vaginal deliveries are safest if the fetal head is at least 2 centimeters below the ischial spines of the pelvis, or well on the way out. Anything higher than that, and I generally couldn't offer a vacuum delivery.

"She's at +1 but she really does move it to +2 with pushing, and I think it will be +2 to 3 very soon. It's just that every time she pushes there's a big deep dip in the fetal heart tracing."

"Does she have an epidural? What's the size of this baby?" I ask.

"Yes. Not big—probably around 3,400 grams."

By this point in our conversation, we have walked the few yards back to the main nursing station. We look up at the monitors, still talking, and see the fetal heart rates on the big screen. Room 4 has just started a big deceleration. Room 4 is Helen's room. The patient isn't pushing and this is still happening.

Helen and I walk quickly to the room; the nurse is already there. We hear the fetal heart rate on the monitor, bump bump bump, 70 beats per minute, far too slow. Without even talking to each other, the nurse in the room starts to work with Helen and me to perform our well-rehearsed list of procedures that can modify the patient's fetal heart tracing: position change, turning off any oxytocin, offering oxygen. The patient is already on her side, not pushing, with oxygen on her face. We ask her to flip to the other side on the off chance that this would help give more blood flow to the uterus. We wrap her arm in a blood pressure cuff and take a measurement; normal.

A quick look at the monitor tells us that the patient isn't having too many contractions; medication to relax her uterus won't help here. And still bump bump bump: the fetal heart rate is in the 70s and not coming up.

I introduce myself very quickly to the patient while putting on gloves and ask if I can examine her. Her eyes wide behind the oxygen mask, she nods. I agree with Helen about the exam: fully dilated, now +2 station, position occiput anterior, minimal caput, adequate pelvis, not huge baby. The epidural seems to be working well, which helps: the patient can tolerate what I would need to do; she can help.

I have just these few seconds to make a decision: can I offer a safe operative delivery, or do we need to head for the operating room right now? In those few seconds, I think: yes, I can do a vacuum delivery; I think it will work. I say this out loud. Bump bump bump, fetal heart rate still in the 70s.

Helen and the nurse and I start calling for various things and for various people, because an intended vacuum delivery requires a lot of help to be safe. Is the patient's bladder empty? An empty bladder is a prerequisite for a vacuum delivery to avoid damage to it. The patient had her bladder emptied less than 10 minutes earlier in anticipation of delivery; no need. Pediatricians available? Yes, they're on their way. Please open an OR for us, just in case? Yes, the nurse manager is aware of the situation and already taking care of it. The delivery table is ready; someone throws a vacuum apparatus on top of the table for me. Bump bump bump, still in the 70s. I don't unwrap the surgical gown or put it on; we don't have time.

I can't tell you what I said to the patient because it was too quick—too much to arrange in too short a time. I probably said something like this: "I'm so sorry to meet you this way. You're very close to hav-

ing this baby, but the baby is showing us a fair amount of stress, so
we have to deliver now. I can help with a vacuum, and at this point, I
think that's safer than trying to do a cesarean, for both you and the
baby. The vacuum has some risks, most of them are minor. The big
deal that you need to know is that if it doesn't work, I think we'll have
to head to the operating room for an emergency cesarean. But I am
going to try this because I think it will work, and I think it's our best
option for right now. You will still need to push very hard; the vacuum shortens this time, but it's still mostly you. Is it okay if I proceed
with the vacuum?"

The patient says: "Yes. Please."

The vacuum available at this hospital is a disposable one; it looks
a bit like a child's bath toy. It has a large white plastic handle with
a pump to initiate and hold vacuum suction. Next to the pump is a
meter that shows the strength of the vacuum suction. Attached to
the dial is a short flexible hose, which blooms into a soft white mush-
room cap, padded inside and sized to fit on a fetal head.

I put the flexible plastic cup on the baby's head, pushing it to the
right position, a few centimeters above the soft spot I can feel in its
skull. This placement means that the correct pull will flex the fetal
head more and present the smallest possible diameter for delivery.
While placing the cup, I make sure that no vaginal tissue is caught
under it, which can cause a very damaging tear. I keep my right hand
on the cup, fingers lying on the fetal head, to make sure my placement doesn't shift; I'm left-handed, so my stronger hand remains on
the vacuum handle, ready to go.

I look up; it has been less than a minute since we made the decision, and already the room is full of people, all there to help. The
pediatricians are in the corner, murmuring and unwrapping equip-

ment. The nurse manager is there and mouths silently to me, "The OR is open if you need it." I nod. The fetal heart rate remains in the 70s, bump bump bump, now for over 4 minutes. A contraction is starting. This is our chance.

Despite her epidural, the patient is aware of her contractions, and she can tell that one is beginning. I lean over the vacuum; I want her to see my face, because we need to act together or this will never work. I say, "It's time. Push, and we'll work together. This needs to be your strongest push ever."

I click up the vacuum until the dial is at the top of the green, the highest safest suction the equipment can provide. With help from her husband on one side and her nurse on the other, the patient draws her legs up even closer to her shoulders, closes her eyes, takes a deep breath, and bears down.

With any operative vaginal delivery, there's no way to know what you are going to get until you start. Sometimes you pull and nothing happens. Sometimes you pull too hard, and the vacuum pops off. If the vacuum pops off three times, most hospital protocols agree: you're done; this vacuum delivery isn't happening; it's time to head to the operating room.

This time, as she bears down and I begin to pull, there is descent of the fetal head, lovely smooth descent, long, controlled descent, answers-to-my-prayers descent. The patient pushes, and I bend my knees slightly as I draw the vacuum toward me, pulling the fetal head down, down under the pubic symphysis. Once that is accomplished, I straighten up to pull the head up up up into the light of our room. Up, up, up, and I am lifting up with my shoulders to bring this baby out and through. As I haul the baby into the world, I can feel in my shoulders and belly that this is happening, this is working, this is the right decision. Everyone in the room can see it too, and it feels like the whole room—me included—is holding our collective breath with the laboring woman.

With the patient's first push, the baby's head comes all the way to her skin edge; with her second push, the head is out. I release the pressure of the vacuum, remove the cup off the baby's head, and throw the vacuum apparatus behind me on the delivery table. The baby turns its head to align with its spine. The baby is catching up to us, completing the normal movements of delivery that we had hurried along.

I am ready for the rest of this delivery to be difficult; a vacuum delivery can increase the risk of a shoulder dystocia, a situation where the baby's head is delivered but the shoulders get stuck, a true obstetric emergency.

"One last push," I tell the patient. "Now this one has to be your strongest push ever." She pushes, and I guide the shoulders down and then up and then out; no shoulder dystocia. I reach for the cord clamps so that I can cut the cord and give the baby to the pediatricians; this is standard procedure after a vacuum delivery, especially if the operative delivery was performed because of concerns for a stressed baby.

But the baby is already crying and moving. The pediatrician has come to my side, and looking at the baby, he sees what I see—the baby's arms and legs flexing, her color pinking up, her ribs not working too hard with each breath. He taps me on the shoulder and says, "That kid is fine. I'll come check her out in 10 minutes, but you can let them be for now." I put the baby right up on her mother's chest, skin to skin, and step back.

I survey the patient: minimal bleeding; the placenta still needs to separate. I will need to inspect the patient for a tear or anything that might need repair. I will need to deliver the placenta. I will need to document everything. But right that second, there is nothing I can or should do. I turn around and plant my sterile gloved hands wide on the delivery table. Trying to let some of the adrenaline of that 4½ minutes crawl down my shoulders and out, I lean over on my arms. I feel like a superhero after she's transformed back to her old, human self. I feel like the Incredible Hulk after he's saved the day: I am still green, but the danger is past, and now I need to become flesh-colored again. I wonder if the Incredible Hulk was also this nauseated and shaky after saving the day. Everything is fine.

Later, when I documented the events, I couldn't remember exactly what I said to the patient before that vacuum delivery. I can tell you that my delivery note says: "Verbal consent obtained." I can tell you that everything I told the patient was the truth and that she agreed to the vacuum; I will also tell you that it was a beautiful vacuum delivery and absolutely the right choice in this situation.

But I think we can also agree that the verbal consent I obtained was not fully informed; there are ways in which, given the pressure the patient was under, it was not really consent. It would have been very hard for her to say no. There was no opportunity to ask questions. My discussion of the risks and benefits and alternatives was extremely abbreviated. Is this fair? Is this the best we can do?

And yet, the opposite—too much information—isn't much better. I worked with one doctor who had a different model for this kind of consent. She had worked in a U.S. military hospital abroad, and there, every patient (most of them soldiers) signed a 30-page consent booklet at the beginning of her pregnancy. It described almost every possible procedure: vacuum delivery, forceps, cesarean delivery, rupture of membranes, fetal scalp electrode, postdelivery emergent hysterectomy—everything. Few of the low-risk, generally healthy military patients would undergo even one of those procedures; nobody would undergo all of them. Everyone got the booklet, and everyone signed it during their prenatal care. Everyone came to L&D already consented for a vacuum delivery. "We had that signed piece of paper for every single person," this doctor said. "It was so much better, you know? I felt so much safer."

Maybe, I thought. But 30 pages? Signed months ago? Consenting for procedures of which most of them would undergo zero, and none of them would undergo all? Is that informed? Is that consent? Or is that a bunch of paper? I know that my colleague felt more covered as a physician—she had written proof that the patients had been counseled, that they had agreed. But how did the patients feel? Neither of us really had any idea.

. . .

THIS PENDULUM, FROM too little consent to too much paperwork that we call consent, is illustrated quite beautifully and frustratingly by the historical and current situation of female sterilization. Often termed "getting your tubes tied," tubal ligation is one of the oldest and most widely used methods of contraception in this country. It can also be a rough and obstructed road for many women.

Despite the availability of multiple other contraceptive methods, tubal ligation is still remarkably in demand. The most requested form of tubal ligation (15 percent in some studies[2]) is postpartum tubal ligation—getting "tubes tied" immediately after a delivery. Postpartum tubal ligation is popular in part because it's a simple surgery, done at the time of an already-expected hospitalization. If a woman undergoes a cesarean delivery, the tubes can be tied, cut, and cauterized during the same surgery. If she's undergone a vaginal delivery, the large size of the recently postpartum uterus allows for a small incision right under the belly button, and both tubes can easily be found, tied, cut, and cauterized.

However, tubal ligation in the United States does not have a benign past. There is a long and shameful history of nonconsensual medical procedures in this country, in particular regarding women's sterilization. Many examples of involuntary or even compulsory sterilization programs have paved the roads of American policy. In the mid-twentieth century, up to 25 to 50 percent of Native American women were regularly sterilized without their consent, often when they were teenagers; many of them didn't know this had been done to them until they unsuccessfully tried to conceive later in life.[3] Similar stories exist with regard to disabled people or those with mental illness.[4] Other racially discriminatory sterilization experiences tied to various eugenics movements litter our history. These programs usually targeted anyone without power: intellectually disabled or mentally ill patients, women of color, or low-income women. Generally, these surgeries occurred not because a patient wasn't capable of consent, but because someone in power—her doctor, her parent, some government official—decided that the world would be better if she did not produce children.

The dramatic rise of sterilization as a popular method of contraception in the United States began in the 1960s and continued into the 1970s. The surgery itself was transformed through the development of new techniques that were safer and easier to utilize. These coincided with the creation of federally funded family planning programs, which subsidized the costs of these surgeries. At that same time, many reports of involuntary sterilization of minority and low-income women emerged. This wasn't the first time this had happened, but this time there was public outcry.

In response, the federal government developed strict regulations regarding consent for sterilization surgeries performed with government funding—which includes any woman on Medicaid or Medicare. These regulations have been in place since 1978, and they require that women who request publicly funded sterilization complete the "Consent to Sterilization" section of the Medicaid Title XIX form. The form must be completed at least 30 days and no more than 180 days before undergoing the sterilization procedure. In addition, a signed copy of the consent form must be available or verified at the time of the procedure. If the woman ends up undergoing emergency abdominal surgery or a premature delivery, the 30-day waiting period may be waived, but even then, at least 72 hours must elapse between the consent and the procedure. If these conditions are not met, the tubal ligation cannot be performed.

It is worth noting that these regulations covering publicly funded sterilization apply to a huge number of women. The relevant population includes anyone covered by Medicaid or Medicare, representing anywhere from 27 to 72 percent of all births in the United States, although the exact rate depends on the state.[5]

Thus, we have an enormous number of women now covered by regulations that have not changed since 1978. These regulations were put in place to protect women, to make sure that all women undergoing sterilization are truly being informed and truly consenting. But the end result, in my experience, is something entirely different, something much less consistent with what consent should be. Now, instead of the consent process protecting a woman, often it obstructs her. That is, most often, what I see in clinical practice is a patient who wants tubal ligation surgery but is not allowed to get it. This happens for a wide variety of reasons, and it happens quite frequently.

The consent form itself, colloquially called "tubal papers," is the first barrier; signing it isn't an easy or short task. It's in complicated language, not easily understood by someone without a high school diploma or without native English. Just filling it out, even with an educated, native English speaker, requires a hefty counseling session, something that could never be accomplished in a typical 15-minute prenatal visit. The ramifications of the surgery need to be reviewed; patients need to know that sterilization is, for all intents and purposes, permanent.[6] This particular counseling remains extremely relevant: many patients think that we can tie their tubes and then just "untie" them if they want another baby. Nope. During tubal ligation, we cut the tubes and stitch them and then cauterize them with electricity. This surgery is for someone who really, really means it when they say they don't want to get pregnant again.

The sterilization consent form also requires that surgical risks be reviewed (though this will occur again when the patient is consented for the actual surgery, a separate consent form) and that the patient receive information about contraceptive alternatives. All of this takes a long time, which is appropriate. But because the counseling is so extensive, "signing tubal papers" usually requires either a separate appointment or a whole separate provider (for example, a clinic social worker). It's an important visit but it's an added task: perhaps a patient has to take another half-day off of work to get this done or pay for a babysitter.

Even when we do manage to get the papers signed, there's the question of timing: that signing needs to happen at least 30 days before a potential delivery but not too early in the pregnancy or we risk it expiring after 180 days. And then—here's the tricky part—that signed paper needs to be produced on the day of delivery so that the surgery can be "confirmed" by the surgeon at the time of the sterilization. So yes, a copy of it needs to come with the patient whose water broke in the grocery store, or the one who started bleeding at home, or the one who got sent straight from clinic for blood pressures in the preeclamptic range. If they don't have the papers in their purse that day, they are completely out of luck. Any snafu with the form creates a situation in which she absolutely, totally will not get her procedure, even if we are already performing her cesarean delivery and she has already undergone the surgical risks involved.

In one clinic where I worked, after too many canceled postpartum tubal ligation surgeries, we started giving people 10 copies of the signed form: "Put it in your purse. Put another copy in your other purse. Give one to your husband and one to your best friend and one to someone else who lives near the hospital." With the advent of electronic medical records (EMR), we can scan the forms into the system. But computers aren't perfect either: I've had those scans go missing or be filed under the wrong date or the wrong patient.

In the end, the regulations that created this consent process for sterilization created a capricious dictatorship. We try to cope; we try to provide for our patients what they want. I've moved cesarean delivery dates purely so that the 30-day requirement be met, medical and obstetric indications permitting, just so that the patient would not have her plans changed in the operating room. Even so, I've had patients sign the forms 29 days prior to their delivery—no tubal ligation. I've had patients sign tubal papers 181 days prior to their delivery—no tubal ligation. I've had patients sign the forms and then lose them—no tubal ligation. I've had patients sign the forms, scan them into the medical record, and then have the medical record lose them—no tubal ligation.

I've even had one patient who brought her forms the day of her surgery, handed them to our doctors to place in the chart, and somehow *we lost them* over the 2 hours that comprised her preoperative care. She handed her papers to the off-going night team at 7 a.m.; when her surgical time rolled around at 9 a.m., none of the day team could find them. I remember ripping up the entire nursing station, lifting up computers that had not been off the desk for years; our intern, God bless him, volunteered to dumpster-dive through the trash bin. In the end, nothing. Nobody could find them. We called our head of labor and delivery and our head of obstetrics for some sort of special permission; but not even our boss or our boss's boss could figure out a way out of the situation: we couldn't do the tubal.[7] Our patient cried with frustration in the preoperative room, and we all wanted to cry with her. In the end, she underwent her cesarean delivery, and her tubes were left alone. If she still wanted sterilization, she would now need to have another surgery to get it with concomitant surgical risks, time off of work, and other challenges. And, of course, if she's one of the many patients who are covered only by emergency Medicaid during pregnancy, then she will somehow need to figure out how to get all this done within the next 6 weeks, before her coverage kicks her off, while recovering from the surgery she already had.

As many as 47 percent of women who request a postpartum tubal ligation do not end up undergoing one in that same pregnancy.[8] The reproductive consequences of the delayed or undone tubal ligation are pretty severe: half of those who never intended to become pregnant again do so, nearly half within a year.[9] Many of the women who are pursuing sterilization have already been failed by other contraceptive options, either because of side effects or limited access or for other reasons. Some of these women have pregnancy-associated illnesses like diabetes and hypertension that make hormonal contraception risky but subsequent pregnancies even riskier. Many of them are not covered by federal (or any) insurance when they're not pregnant or immediately postpartum, so they leave the hospital without their tubal ligation; they go home without contraception or any medical care. They return, often pregnant, and often entering the pregnancy sicker and at higher risk, and all that risk in the setting of a pregnancy they didn't want. All this because of a missing piece of paper.

For women on private insurance—generally higher-income women—the experience is completely different. They can sign their own piece of paper; they can sign it on the morning of the surgery or whenever they damn well please.

This federal response to abuse, this cure for involuntary sterilization, has inadvertently created a two-tier system: one where we believe women who say what they want and one where we don't.

Long ago, sterilization consent was far too little of a process with far too little information. That led to some very, very bad things. Now it's a process unchanged since 1978; it's far too much of a process, far too restrictive, and that itself is leading to some other very bad things, but only for some people. That's how it goes with consent: there's a million ways to do it wrong, and only a few ways to do it right.

. . .

SOMETIMES CONSENT CAN be inadequate, even before it's over-informed or underinformed; just the fact that consent is required for a particular situation can be both revelatory and disturbing. Consider normal labor and normal vaginal delivery. I've now read multiple very angry articles about the lack of consent for labor and for a spontaneous vaginal delivery; many of these articles were written by women who started looking into this issue because they felt incredibly under-counseled and underinformed before their difficult vaginal deliveries:[10] "Shouldn't someone have warned me about how hard this would be? The bleeding, and the pain, and the fact that I ended up at a cesarean delivery anyway? Where was my consent process for my labor? Where was my consent process that allowed my vaginal delivery?"

I always have a profound and somewhat violent negative reaction to these requests for consent for a vaginal delivery. On the one hand, I agree that the education portion of their program was inadequate; anyone and everyone should know anything and everything that they want to about their upcoming labor. The source of this information might need to be your doctor or perhaps a doula; or some of this may be a job for a really excellent library.

But I fundamentally disagree with their demand for consent for labor and delivery. It makes me angry to consider a consent process, mediated by a physician, for something that is fundamentally natural. Labor is not pathology; delivery is not a disease. Labor and delivery is something a body is doing—a powerful, independent, adult human body—by itself. In fact, part of why I have such a strong reaction to this idea is that women fought for years, decades, and even centuries to assert their own control over this bodily function. And if a consent process for normal labor and vaginal delivery were initiated, what would the woman be agreeing to when she signed such a paper? She would be agreeing to allow what is happening to continue to happen; that is, she would be agreeing to allow a physician to *not* perform a cesarean delivery. The default option, then, as implied by this consent process, is that the cesarean delivery would be safer or easier (and this is manifestly not true; see Chapter 6).

Finally, the reality of pregnancy, labor, and delivery is that these are all bodily functions. We don't sign a consent for other bodily functions—burping or defecating or vomiting—though they may not be pleasant and even on occasion may lead to complications. It would be absurd to sign consent for those things: to whom would we be granting consent? This action is not being done to a woman's body by another. Similarly, labor and delivery involves a woman's body doing something for herself and to herself. (This is not just the way I feel. Aaron Caughey, chair of the Department of Obstetrics and Gynecology at Oregon Health & Science University and vice chair of the ACOG Committee on Practice Bulletins-Obstetrics, has stated: "Informed consent is an ethical concept designed to respect patients' moral right to bodily integrity by protecting them from unwanted medical treatment or intervention, but giving birth vaginally is a natural physiologic process that by definition is not medical treatment"[11]).

To me, that's the worst and most paternalistic aspect of offering "consent" for labor and delivery. Signing consent for something your body *does*, a function your body performs, is pretending that natural labor is something that someone else does to you. It is pretending that someone else is in charge. It is the relinquishing of agency over your own body and what it is doing—agency that women have fought for years to establish.

But even this opposition to the idea of consent for vaginal delivery changes with context. It becomes completely different when someone goes into labor who has undergone a cesarean delivery in the past. In that situation, when a woman with a scar on her uterus shows up in labor (for TOLAC; see Chapter 6), most facilities will make sure that she signs consent to allow them ("allow them") to continue labor. The signed consent says that the patient was counseled about the risks of uterine rupture, that she was offered a cesarean and declined.

When we are discussing a body that has previously undergone cesarean, our medical and legal systems have decided that now there *is* a need for consent. With this change, those systems are saying that labor and delivery is not the default; a repeat cesarean is the default, and we are asking for the patient's permission to not perform the default treatment. What your body is doing, that consent form implies, may be natural, but it's not *only* natural. Because of that previous intervention, labor and delivery is now, somehow, not regarded as the healthy physiology of a body functioning as it should; it is somehow, now, under the jurisdiction of someone else.

It seems that this is how the idea of consent might currently be utilized: the need for consent written in the history of your body. If your uterus is unscarred, then labor and delivery doesn't need consent. But if you have a scar on your uterus, then the very existence of the consent form states that doctors cannot be uninvolved in your subsequent labor even if it is spontaneous; even if it is a bodily function. Because surgery was performed years ago, because that surgery is still in your body, we need consent now: consent to not operate, permission for an un-surgery. In this example, given that the past is not modifiable, the consent form is less of a consent for action than for a consent for inaction. It may be that as much as it is a consent, it's also a signature that serves as a paper trail to offload provider responsibility.

Here's another example of a similar kind of "consent," one of my least favorite: several institutions, in the wake of the high American prevalence of obese patients, have started requiring morbidly obese patients to sign a special consent form. The consent says that the patient understands that because of her weight, we may not be able to perform a cesarean delivery as quickly; that any surgery may involve more complications; that her care is influenced in many ways by her weight; and that therefore her expectations may need to be different.

This is why I really dislike this particular example of consent: How, precisely, is this a consent form? And consent for what—for daring to live as a fat[12] person? What is her alternative? To leave the hospital? To start a weight loss regimen in the hallway while awaiting her bed on labor and delivery? To spontaneously combust prior to finishing her pregnancy? I understand that the consent is supposed to attest that these issues were considered and discussed; I also understand that without this process, these issues are hard to raise and are often ignored. But to call this process "consent" and have the patient sign a form for something so unmodifiable just feels mean. What have we accomplished by having a patient sign that she will accept a lower standard of care? What is she consenting to, besides acknowledging our own discrimination and her awareness of inferior treatment?

Even the more traditional consent for straightforward procedures is a minefield. For example, when consenting a patient for any surgery, what amount of dread is appropriate to bring to the occasion? It seems appropriate to mention risk of infection (2 to 16 percent of cesarean deliveries) and bleeding requiring transfusion (2 to 4 percent of cesarean deliveries) and damage to adjacent organs (0.2 to 0.5 percent).[13] Should the consent form include hysterectomy? It's something that does occur, though it's relatively rare: 0.24 to 8.7 per 1,000 deliveries.[14] But when an unplanned peripartum hysterectomy occurs, it can be a fundamentally life-altering complication, ending childbearing. Should a patient be told that, well, it can happen, though it probably won't today? And if we're mentioning rare but devastating complications, then let's discuss maternal death. Death is potentially a complication of cesarean delivery, and it is a possibility; it's a higher possibility than it should be, especially in the United States (see Chapter 10). But in absolute numbers, this woman's chance of death from this cesarean is vanishingly low.

Is it fair to add "risk of death" to a consent form for a cesarean delivery? At some point, the damage the anxiety provokes outdoes any minor advantage of being informed about all possible surgical results. Even when we emphasize numbers and say "this complication is exceedingly rare," it can still be misleading. By including rare and catastrophic scenarios, they become present. Their very existence, even if quantified, makes them seem not only possible but probable. Thus, a patient who needs a cesarean delivery for a placenta previa may think, "Well, I'm going to bleed to death anyway; I'd rather do it outside the operating room." But in fact, her cesarean delivery is many, many times safer for her, and by not curating the information we're giving her, we're misleading her just as much as we would by omitting information.

Finally, when we add rare complications like "death" to consent forms, I'm not sure we're doing so to fully inform a patient, though that's putatively the point. When we add such an extreme risk to a consent form, it often seems, as in the example with obesity consent, that this consent process is another way to assign to the patient the moral responsibility for any dread possibility that might occur. If adding rare or nonmodifiable possibilities doesn't change anything about the surgery or the patient's choice, then why is it on a consent

form? Such information on a consent form is unnecessarily anxiety provoking and present to benefit the physician and the medical
system; it creates the illusion that the physician is no longer under
obligation: "I told her it could happen! She signed the paper!" But at
what point is this just threatening a patient?

. . .

INFORMED CONSENT IS a mess, then, and almost impossible to
do correctly. But what would be the right way? How can we fix this?

The right way is to acknowledge that patient consent isn't a form;
it's not a signed piece of paper. Real consent is an undertaking; it's a
discussion; it's the amorphous process by which a patient transmits
what she wants and needs and prioritizes and the medical establishment communicates back what it has to offer and at what cost.
Informed consent is a relationship.

ACOG itself devotes an entire document to this topic and says:

> A signed consent document, however, does not ensure that the
> process of informed consent has taken place in a meaningful
> way or that the ethical requirements have been met. . . . To focus
> on the importance of communication for the implementation of
> an ethical doctrine of informed consent is, then, to underline
> the fact that informed consent involves a process. There is a pro-
> cess of communication that leads to initial consent (or refusal to
> consent) and that can make possible appropriate ongoing deci-
> sion making.[15]

In my experience, this kind of consent is the hardest to do; it's
a hard skill set to learn. It's something that I wasn't great at when I

became a doctor and even for many years afterward; I like to think I'm a lot better at it now.

For a medical practitioner, real consent involves more than just knowledge and more than just capability. It involves a willingness to be rejected and an aversion to defensiveness. Real consent involves setting forward your gifts: your scientific knowledge, your years of training, your 2 a.m. exhausted presence. It involves laying those gifts out before a patient, with the full willingness and knowledge that they may be accepted, declined, or something in between.

Real consent requires everything that goes on the signed form. It still requires the complete medical knowledge to know what to offer and what information to provide. It requires experience to apply that knowledge to an appropriate patient. But more than that, it requires whatever skill allows us to know that the person before us is both very much like us and yet entirely different, with priorities and challenges and the right to make decisions that we think are explicable or not, decisions that are smart or wrong or stupid or even harmful. I don't know what we call that skill. Empathy? Compassion? Humility?

Let me end with the story of a particular type of consent—the signing of an "Against Medical Advice" (AMA) form. A patient who doesn't want an intervention that doctors recommend—a surgery, a medication, an inpatient hospital stay—will often be asked ("asked," not ordered) to sign a paper that she is refusing what we, the medical establishment, think is best.

. . .

AMALIA POLLEY WAS pregnant with her third baby. She had a 6-year-old son and a 4-year-old daughter at home and had uncomplicated term pregnancies with both of them. Somehow, during this pregnancy, her water broke much too early and she came in to our triage unit at 24 weeks pregnant. The first few days of this hospital- ization were a crisis, as is usual with this kind of event. We talked endlessly about periviable birth (see Chapter 5) and death and what might happen if she went into labor. We gave her antibiotics. We recruited experts from the neonatology ICU to come and talk with her about outcomes. We told her that she would likely go into labor within 2 weeks; that's what the data showed. We recommended that she stay in the hospital until she delivered. This situation can change fast, we said. Sometimes you get an infection; sometimes you go into labor; sometimes you start to bleed. We keep all our patients with ruptured membranes in the hospital. If we're lucky we get weeks; if we're luckier we get months. Boredom, we said, isn't the worst thing.

A day passed, and Amalia received her second steroid shot. A week passed, and she finished the course of antibiotics designed to keep her uterus quiet and calm. Two weeks passed, and she was still pregnant. Every day we put her and her baby on the monitor, and every day her uterus was calm and the fetal heart rate looked great. Twice a week, we sent her for ultrasounds, which always showed low fluid but some fluid. And every 2 weeks, we measured the fetal growth. The baby always looked healthy and was grow- ing well. Amalia's pregnancy was no longer periviable; our mode of care switched, imperceptibly, from urgent-crisis mode to long- term-management mode.

For the first week, Amalia was just grateful to still be pregnant; grateful to be in the hospital; grateful to still require care. But even in those first few days, the burden of caring for her other kids weighed on her. In the mornings, I would often find her in tears. "I'm missing my kids today," she would say. She told us she was lucky in that she did have a husband she trusted who was "great with the little one." The problem was that her husband worked in construction, and if he didn't work, he couldn't earn money.

For the first few days or even a week of Amalia's hospitalization, relatives pitched in; then some people from the church. After 2 weeks, Amalia's husband got fired. Now he was able to stay home with the kids, but the worries about childcare were replaced with worries about money. After a month, Amalia's family had no money for rent and was worried about losing their apartment.

Our team offered what it could. We had a social worker meet with her to identify what resources were available, but the truth is that none were. I offered to write any doctor's note necessary to anyone: Her husband's boss? The landlord? But Amalia's husband didn't work for a big company; his job didn't need to comply with FMLA (the Family and Medical Leave Act). Their apartment landlord didn't care about my note or Amalia's health. So I shouldn't have been surprised when one day, after 4½ weeks of hospitalization, Amalia told me she needed to go home.

A long time ago, my counseling for someone in this situation, signing out of the hospital "against medical advice" (AMA) was harsh. As a new doctor, I would have told her everything my superiors told me: that her baby could die; that she could die. This is all true; such incidences do occur (see Chapter 10). It was, in fact, riskier for Amalia to be at home.

But the counseling for AMA can go beyond what is necessary just to explain the risks of leaving our treatment. I used to overhear some doctors telling patients that if they signed out against medical advice, they would be liable for the entire hospitalization, that somehow their AMA signature would prove to the insurance company that they didn't deserve any of the care they received. This is false, and I corrected it every time I heard it—but it was an effective financial threat. It meant that patients, facing a multi-thousand-dollar debt from their days or weeks of hospitalization, would stay with us, often against their own best interests.

That financial threat was a lie, but the militancy and anger behind it was, I think, genuine. The AMA process is supposedly about what a patient's best interests are, but there's something else there that is not addressed: an anger, a defensiveness, a rejection. In theory, we provide counseling for a patient who wants to sign out AMA because we want her to have what's best for her: we want her to stay, to let us take care of her, to let us provide all the answers that our years of training can give. We are willing to spend a million dollars on her; we are happy to do that. How can she reject this gift? That's the hostility that we haven't addressed, the anger of the spurned; and it's that hostility that makes the AMA process more hostile and less functional than it otherwise could be.

And there's also pride, I think: a doctor wants to give the correct care, the care that was the right answer on the exam question. Giving different care can be wrong; it can cause harm. But it can also feel like being asked to be the doctor who didn't know the right answer on the exam, and we all want to be prouder of our work than that. If the right antibiotic is intravenous, I don't want to be forced into using an oral formulation that she can take at home; if the right answer is surgery, how can I let this patient leave my hands without it? This pride, too, I think, lay under the AMA process.

For these reasons, or perhaps for others, AMA used to be a dead end, a parting of ways marked by this disagreement between a medical institution and a patient. If the patient wouldn't heed the counseling, if the patient insisted on signing out AMA, death, dismemberment, bankruptcy be damned, then that was the end. The form would be signed, and the patient would walk out of the hospital and essentially off a cliff: no doctor, no prescriptions, no appointments, no plan. The way AMA used to be was all or nothing: if you won't accept all our gifts, you can't have any of them. We provide optimal care as we see it, or we provide no care at all. Patient rejection led to total provider abandonment.

But of course, from Amalia's perspective, it wasn't that she didn't want to be safe; it wasn't even that she didn't want to listen to her medical team. From what Amalia could see, whatever she may lose by leaving the hospital, she was losing more by staying. From her perspective, signing an AMA rife with medical and financial threats isn't her doctors trying to do what's best for her but her doctors trying to keep her in their control. She was in the midst of a complicated and challenging life, and only she knew what was best for her.

How can we meet her, and other patients like her, there? How can we ask her to sign AMA in a way that is informed but also consent, a way that acknowledges her larger life, her ability to make choices?

There is a better way, and many of us are getting there. That is, we sign an AMA form with a patient—and we still make it clear that this is not what we recommend. But once that AMA form is signed, we stop and think. Plan A doesn't work for everyone, but nobody's off the hook. What can we do that would be a decent plan B that would meet the patient's priorities and provide some level of care, even if not optimal? What about a plan C? It's a process and a continuing relationship, and it's never over and it's never straightforward. This isn't just good medicine; it's good care, and it's on its way to becoming a new standard.

That day when Amalia told the resident she wanted to sign out AMA after a full month of inpatient care, the resident balked. The resident told Amalia everything she had been taught about our plan A: that the baby could die; that Amalia could die. Amalia was firm: she knew that; she had been told this, many times. However, Amalia was going to leave, the sooner the better, that day. I was summoned, as the attending on call, to argue with her, to supervise the signing of the AMA.

I knew Amalia well; after more than a month in the hospital, she knew all the doctors and nurses. I walked in, and Amalia said, "Doctor, I know I'm allowed to leave. This isn't jail."

"You're right," I said. "This isn't jail. You can leave whenever you want to."

"I am leaving today."

"I know you are. Listen, Ms. Polley, I know the other doctor told you that you could die and that the baby could die. Those are true, though rare, and I do think that it's safer for you to be here. Is there any way we could help you stay?"

Amalia shook her head: "My kids need me, and my husband needs me. We can't lose our place."

"I understand," I said. "If you decide to leave, I'm going to ask you to sign this form, because, as we've already explained, you're leaving against medical advice—against what we think is best. But that doesn't mean it's the end of us taking care of you; it just means we need to figure out what we can manage."

Together we hashed out a calendar. Amalia said she could come once a week for fetal monitoring if she came in the morning when the kids were at school. I pushed her a little bit: could she manage twice a week and get an ultrasound and a blood test? She thought she could.

"At least this week," I said, "your first week home. I just want to make sure we're not missing anything. If you can come on Tuesday, I'll see you myself: I'll be staffing the ultrasound unit."

I reviewed with her that things could change very quickly: if she developed a fever, if she felt contractions, if she started bleeding, or if she felt decreased fetal movement, then she needed to make her way to the hospital right away. "Please line up someone who can take the kids quickly, in an emergency," I said. "I hope it won't happen, but let's make a plan now so that you can be here as quickly as possible when you need to be. If you find a way to have things taken care of so that you can be here in the hospital, please come back: we'd love to take you back whenever we can, for whatever time we get."

This is the new "against medical advice" consent; it is conducted, paradoxically, with a ton of medical advice. Amalia was leaving; she was rejecting what I had. But if we did this right, she was not leaving my care, and she was not falling off a cliff. Instead, she was traveling down her road, equipped with as much of our wisdom and resources as we could load up. This is real, true medical consent: it is where perfect laboratory knowledge meets an imperfect real life. It is where Amalia's ruptured membranes met her two young children and her husband's job. It is a process of getting what we can, for as many as we can, together.

This kind of incremental, iterative AMA has become policy at many hospitals, and I think it is a new model for what real true consent can be. The new AMA process still involves a piece of paper, and that piece of paper gets signed; but the consent is bigger and broader than that. The consent process here is a communication, but not a one-time communication; it's a relationship, a bargain, a contract that can be made and remade as the patient and doctor move through changing circumstances. This consent is an ongoing experience, not of offering and rejection, but of offering and reoffering and acceptance, then reassessing and starting all over again. It is exhausting, and it is time-consuming, and it works.

Amalia signed the AMA paper. She packed up her small room, and by lunchtime, Amalia was ready to walk out the door to her waiting husband and kids. "See you Tuesday," she said.

I laughed: "Yep, see you Tuesday, unless you need to come back before then. We'll take you back anytime, you know."

"I know," she said. "But I'll see you on Tuesday."

9.

Medical Systems and Home Birth

How Institutions Save You or Fail You or Both

The way most of us have babies today differs from the way most of our ancestors did. I don't just mean that we've gotten rid of the cave or the wet-nurse or the high neonatal death rate. Many of the ways that childbirth has changed have to do with advances in technology or advances in expectations, and many of those changes have been created by and within the organizations that care for us during these times in our lives.

These days, having a baby isn't just about contractions or blood; it's not even just about the clinic visits or the ultrasounds or amniotic fluid. It's also about the waiting and the paperwork and the hospital bracelet and the medical record number. For many of us (though not, of course, for all of us), pregnancy is our first journey deep into the modern medical system. Pregnancy becomes an experience in which encountering the medical system means taking your individual particular body, which has always housed your individual particular self, and sometimes, for the first time, having that body be subjected to paperwork and protocols; having it tagged, scanned, and in every way made into a datum.

When I say the modern medical system, I include, of course, the clinic office where prenatal visits happen and the hospital where patients get admitted and deliver. But I also mean the parts you don't see: the laboratory and the insurance company and the salespeople at the start-up medical device company. And I mean the *institution* of the modern medical system: the protocols and the administration and the computer systems and the bureaucracy. All of it makes up the complicated, multitentacled monster whose business is caring for the human body in sickness and in health.

The shock that most of us feel after delivery is in large part from the pregnancy, the labor, and the completely absorbing responsibility of caring for a new vulnerable human. But part of that shock also, I think, sometimes originates in the encounter with the giant regimented medical system and what it makes of us. There's a jolt in realizing how little we knew and how much, without realizing it, we expected it to be different—and even more, how much power we gave up—was it necessary to give it up?—over our own body to that system.

. . .

MEDICAL SYSTEMS ARE huge, and for the most part, there's a good reason for that. The modern medical system was built to treat the sickest possible patient.

That means that what the modern medical system does really, really well is acute complicated care. If you have chest pain while in the food court at the mall, and the EMTs find that the electrocardiogram is concerning for a massive heart attack, you can watch that mechanism go into action as you ride in the ambulance. Before you can take a deep breath, you will have been assessed by at least three doctors and five nurses, taken to a catheterization lab that looks like something out of the Jetsons, and had your coronary vessels popped open by some of the most modern and least invasive technology that has ever existed. The procedure will be safe, extremely effective, and incredibly fast: the standard of care is 90 minutes to opening up the arteries that feed the heart from the minute the wheel of your stretcher bumps over the threshold.[1]

I once went to see a patient in the postanesthesia care unit (PACU) at 6:30 a.m.; she had undergone emergency surgery overnight and would be ready to go up to a room soon. Next to her bed, I found her husband openmouthed. He was looking at the people walking in: initially a trickle and then a stream; in the end, something close to a couple of hundred people, all in identical scrubs. Each of them walked in, took a look at the large assignment board behind the main desk, and walked purposefully away, staffing the 20 operating rooms of this large hospital for a typical weekday. By 6:45 a.m., the large room was buzzing, much like a beehive, as the day team streamed in, taking over from the smaller night crew and preparing for a busy day of surgeries. People walked back and forth with trays of sterilized equipment; beeping carts went by with oxygen bottles and large containers of mysterious substances. Some of the people in scrubs carried enormous tool cases; others were carefully carrying just a small vial (medications? tissue sample?); others wore glasses with colored lenses in preparation for laser surgery.

The patient herself was resting with her eyes closed, but her husband was staring in awe and wonderment. "I've never seen anything like this outside the military," he said. "It's so . . . organized."

In the obstetric world, that organization of this medical system means that if a 36-week pregnant woman walks into a major medical institution bleeding, that system will have her intravenous line in place, labs drawn and on the way to the laboratory, and an anesthesiologist starting her sedation, all within 15 minutes. At the same time, a nurse will be finishing her prep for surgery and the operating room team will have all the necessary instruments sterilized, counted, and ready to go. I can deliver that baby within 2 minutes after that, almost every time; by then, the neonatology team will be in the room, ready with their own equipment to resuscitate that baby. To do that requires a cast of thousands and a level of chronic readiness that is impossible for any individual doctor or department to maintain.

In my experience, that's what the large medical system is designed for: the top level of what people need, the highest of acuity, the uppermost common denominator. But this is what, in the end, thankfully, few people need. What about what most people need, most of the time? What about health care that is less urgent but no less necessary?

The modern medical system is like a tank: it is large; it is powerful; it can save lives. But it is also heavy and very difficult to turn around, which means that it can run right over those very same people.

I didn't remind that husband in the PACU, in awe of our efficiency, of his wife's 6 hours in the emergency department, most of the time waiting for an operating room. I didn't tell him how I had to argue to get the anesthesiologist to allow the case to be handled during the night ("Honestly, is it really a level 4 case? Can't she wait until the morning?") and then how I had to have the same argument again with the nursing staff. I didn't discuss how, once we started, the instrument we had requested was not in the room, and there was a 10-minute surgical delay while it was searched for. Nobody died; nobody was really in danger. But getting that organized care wasn't efficient, and it wasn't beautiful. And it wasn't an unusual kind of inefficiency or ugliness; it's what we see much of the time.

The system can, however, have inefficiencies that run the gamut from marginally to profoundly damaging—even, rarely, life-threatening.

. . .

AYO AFOLABE CAME to our office for a consult because of a prior preterm birth. Women who have one preterm birth are at higher risk for another. Ayo had her first baby extremely early—27 weeks—and although the little girl was overall doing well, she had had a rocky course in the NICU, spending almost three months there, with multiple complications resulting from her prematurity. The little girl was now an active 4-year-old with vision problems, and she received some physical therapy services. She was talking but late; it was too early to tell what kind of help she would need in school. But she ran around our clinic and scribbled easily with crayons, and aside from her tiny size and large turquoise glasses, she looked like any other toddler.

Ayo was pregnant again, and she knew she was supposed to come see the high-risk doctors. In the past, we had little to do for patients likes this, but within the last decade, a new treatment has been shown to be effective. Weekly progesterone injections have been shown to reduce the incidence of recurrent preterm births.

These injections are not easy. They are required weekly, and they are intramuscular: they go deep in the muscle of the arm or the thigh, like a flu shot. This means that they hurt a lot; it also means that it's not something that most women can easily learn to do on themselves (as opposed to the subcutaneous injections of medications like insulin). These injections have associated risks such as bleeding or infection if performed improperly. And these injections are time-sensitive: to be most effective, they need to be started relatively early in pregnancy, somewhere around 16 to 20 weeks.[2]

Ayo knew this. And Ayo was smart; after her last delivery, someone had told her that she would need to see a high-risk pregnancy doctor early in pregnancy, and she remembered that. Ayo tried to follow those instructions. But when she called the MFM clinic, the staff informed her that she could not be seen there until she had a referral from her primary prenatal care provider. When she called the primary prenatal care office, that staff told her that they could not issue a referral without seeing her at a first prenatal appointment. Could she make an appointment to get that? Well, the prenatal clinic said, eventually. They also had a rule that a patient had to have evidence of a pregnancy with a fetal heartbeat, usually on ultrasound, prior to being able to make the appointment.

Each of these rules were made for a good reason: when the MFM clinic allowed for direct appointments, we were swamped with patients whose needs could have been met by an OBGYN provider, and the patients who really did need the higher level of consultation weren't able to get to us. The prenatal clinic receives an enormous number of requests for an initial prenatal visit, and initial prenatal visits are high-resource visits, taking 45 minutes to an hour. Given that the early miscarriage rate is so high—somewhere between 25 and 30 percent—many of those appointments would sit unused (that is, until the fetal heartbeat policy was implemented), while other

patients waited months for the next available appointment. Generally, it is good medicine for a health care provider to actually meet
and see a patient before deciding on a course of care, including issu-
ing a referral to MFM. The administrative higher-ups made these
rules for good reasons. All these good reasons, however, ended up
being bad rules for Ayo.

Ayo eventually navigated all of this and ended up at the MFM
clinic by about 15 weeks gestation. In a regular system, with regular medications, getting her progesterone started by 16 to 20 weeks
gestation wouldn't be an issue. But the medication that Ayo needed,
17-hydroxyprogesterone caproate, was phenomenally expensive the
first few years it was marketed for the prevention of recurrent preterm
birth. Although the medication itself was an old chemical—it's just a
version of synthetic progesterone—for a series of complicated financial and regulatory reasons, at that time the medication was essentially only available under the brand name Makena.[3] Makena was
available from only one drug manufacturer, at the jaw-dropping
price of approximately $1,440 per injection, or approximately $6,500
per month. There was a compounded drug available as the closest,
less expensive option; but at the time, compounded medications
were frowned on by the FDA after a series of infections (unrelated to
obstetrics) and were therefore hard to find and also frequently not
covered by insurance.

Ayo was covered by public insurance for her pregnancy, as are
almost half of pregnancies in the United States.[4] Her insurance company, steward of taxpayer money as it was, was reluctant to provide
this costly medication until medical necessity was proved.

There was a special form to fill out on a website, all of it well
beyond Ayo's capabilities. In fact, it was so far beyond the capabili-

ties of any untrained individual that our clinic ultimately assigned a
nurse to these requests for several hours per week. The clinic did this
despite the fact that the nursing time was not something we could
bill for; but if we didn't have a medically savvy staffer devote hours
to these requests, they didn't happen.

Even with the nurse on the case, when we received an initial
answer from the insurance company, it wasn't great news: the medicine would be partially covered, but Ayo would have to pay up front
and then get reimbursed. Ayo would have to pay for the whole bot-
tle—$6,500 worth of medication—in order to start. Ayo was now 16
weeks pregnant.

Ayo heard this number and laughed out loud. She worked as a
home health aide, and that money represented almost two months'
salary. There was absolutely no way for her to amass that kind of
cash or credit and then wait for some unclear amount of reimbursement at some unclear future time.

The clinic staff sent in an appeal to the insurance company; Ayo
went into the Medicaid office. In the end, Ayo switched from one
public insurance company to another that had a more liberal policy
regarding Makena reimbursement. The request was then resubmit-
ted, this time getting approval. Ayo was now 19 weeks pregnant.

So much for the medication. But how would the medication get
into Ayo's body? The insurance company had approved the enormous expenditure of the progesterone itself but had not approved
injection services.

Because the intramuscular injections were difficult for a patient
to do on her own, most insurance companies approved a weekly
visit from a nurse along with the Makena. Ayo's insurance company
had not moved quickly on that aspect. Her remaining option was to

come to the clinic once a week and have our nursing staff administer the injection.

The clinic tried to make this relatively easy on Ayo; we scheduled these visits as unbilled nursing visits. But anything that happens within the clinic itself is still subject to the systems of the clinic itself: thus, our electronic medical system required that Ayo be registered at the front desk and wait for an available nurse. And to actually give the injection, the nurse would still need an order in the computer system, so a doctor would have to be hunted down and begged. All of this took time. Ayo was already over 20 weeks gestational age; it wasn't clear the medicine would be helpful by this point. Ayo also had an hourly job and a special-needs child, so she came to an injection visit once, I think, or perhaps twice. But both times the travel plus the injection visit ate up over 2 hours of her work time. Ayo couldn't maintain this schedule, and she never came in for injections again.

Ayo still came to all her doctor appointments and to her ultrasounds, despite what they cost her in time and money. She often brought her daughter, tiny and in constant motion.

Ayo was still smart. She knew to come to the hospital right away if she had contractions. At 28 weeks, just 1 week after her prior delivery, she came in with contractions and was found to be 2 centimeters dilated. We admitted her, gave her steroids, and stopped her contractions successfully for 48 hours. Ayo was stable for 1 day after that, and then she went into unstoppable preterm labor and delivered an almost 29-week baby, weighing a little over 2 pounds. The baby went right to the NICU and would likely be there until Ayo's due date.

Was this preterm birth preventable?

I don't know. But maybe.

In the end, intramuscular progesterone doesn't prevent every preterm birth; it only cuts the rate by about a third.[5] But Ayo didn't get her progesterone, so she had all of that risk instead of just some of the risk. I don't know if she would have ended up in the lucky percent or the unlucky percent. I do know that at Ayo's postpartum visit, it was hard to look her in the eyes.

Ayo's need for progesterone existed at the intersection of several different threads of the modern medical system: pharmaceutical companies, insurance companies, and outpatient clinics. It existed at the intersection of clerks, pharmacists, nurses and doctors. And right there, at the center of that complicated weave devoted to medical care, there was a big progesterone-shaped hole, and Ayo's care fell right through it.

All of these systems had technically done their jobs; all the forms got filled out, and all the filled-out forms were addressed in a relatively timely fashion. But there was no job that was related to treating Ayo as an individual case with an urgent, proven need; none of the forms was devoted to optimizing her particular, individual outcome. All the rules were followed, but nobody looked at Ayo and said, "She is suffering; this will end badly; let's do it another way." And here is the thing about large systems: even if somebody had, such is the nature of systems that there are few people who would have had the power to overrule the protocols, to spend that money, to get Ayo what she really needed when she really needed it.

Every part of the medical system that failed Ayo had rules: the clinic, the pharmacy, the insurance company. Those rules were generally put into place for good reasons. I think we would all agree that it is reasonable to review spending almost $7,000 per month for medication on the taxpayer's dime.

But that's the very small picture. When we back out just a bit, we realize that the taxpayer is paying anyway. Ayo and her baby are both still on Medicaid. Ayo's daughter's NICU time cost somewhere between $1,000 and $3,000 per day. Per day. For three months. Anyone can do that math and figure out that we didn't save any money.

Then there are the lifelong costs that Ayo's daughter will incur from her preterm birth—eyeglasses, physical therapy, special education—all interventions she's much more likely to need because of her extreme preterm birth, some of them perhaps for the rest of her life. Prenatal interventions are satisfying, not just on a personal level but also in the kind of dry cost-benefit analyses that builds public health policy. Because even a small expense saved early enough leads to exponential savings throughout a life; so almost all prenatal interventions are worthwhile.

In actuality, the lack of progesterone was expensive for Ayo herself. I don't just mean in suffering or lost work or years of trekking to specialist appointments or her lost dreams of returning to college, though those are all true. I mean that despite the many news outlets that may tell you that Ayo is a tax-sucking, anchor-baby-having leech on society, Ayo is a taxpayer. She would probably pay more taxes if she earned more, but she can't earn more while caring for one and now likely two special-needs children. That's another way that preterm birth costs us all money, for those doing the math.

The money, of course, pales in comparison with other things, like suffering and pain and fear and preterm-baby brain damage. But for those who merely want a spreadsheet, the numbers are pretty damning on their own. This was stupid and expensive, it turns out, not just for Ayo but for you and me, because we are part of this society that benefits when Ayo and her baby are healthy and productive.

A large part of what went wrong with Ayo has to do with what a medical system is. A medical system is an industry in which the basic unit of trade is the health of the human body. It's our elemental standard, our economic widget.[6] As a system, most of what is achieved is by making every single widget exactly the same.

Each human is an individual; our bodies are no less idiosyncratic and impossible to reproduce than our personalities. But in a system in charge of moving bodies, we end up treating them as the same. We standardize you, your body, the temple of your soul, the one with the dimple and the left butt cheek freckle and the weird click behind your right knee. And if you or your body doesn't fit into that system, well, it's usually not the system that's going to be forced to change.

I know a woman named Joanna; she has a chronic medical condition that requires respiratory support; she has a permanent tracheostomy and intermittently uses a ventilator to breathe, even when she's out and about. She's had this progressive condition since childhood, and she is never going to get better. The trach and vent setup that she has is one that she arrived at over time to maximize her mobility and quality of life. Joanna needs the vent to breathe; without it, she will die. But she has managed her vent herself for decades, since she was a kid, with the goal of living as normal a life as possible—teaching herself to talk despite a tracheostomy, to function, to attend college and ultimately graduate school. That vent is set up for her particular needs: it allows her to be mobile and independent and as free as possible.

One day Joanna ended up in the hospital, as is not infrequent for people with chronic medical conditions. In this hospital, the staff did not want Joanna to use her vent. The goal of that unit was rehabilitation—to "wean" every patient until they didn't need a vent anymore. Because of that, the vent they utilized was a nonmobile kind; it was attached to the wall. They wanted her to use that vent or none at all. They didn't feel that she could use hers because they didn't have certified personnel to deal with it. So far, understandable: we can all understand why a hospital would pick a ventilator that works for their patient population and why that hospital shouldn't administer a medical device without credentialed personnel.

But Joanna wasn't recovering from a stroke or a car accident; this was her forever body, with its chronic need for a vent. "Weaning" was never going to be a possibility, or a goal, for Joanna.

In the end, during her hospital stay, Joanna ended up with this choice: use the hospital ventilator or no ventilator at all. The hospital provided and maintained their ventilator, but their machine could only be used while Joanna was stuck in bed. This machine was terrifying to Joanna, who had worked hard to be as mobile as possible and was frightened of getting stuck in that bed forever. So Joanna would try to walk a bit, attempting to maintain her mobility, without the ventilator; but without the ventilator, even a small walk was fatiguing and incapacitating, as Joanna knew it would be, as she had told them it would be. Joanna would end up exhausted, sicker, and hooked up to their ventilator—stuck in bed. She might then get a bit better and try to walk again, repeating the cycle again and again. During her weeks in the hospital. Joanna would get sicker, so they could make her "better" on their machine, then sicker, then "better," until she finally got out of there and got her own ventilator back.

All of those decisions may be understandable, and even wise, on their own. The hospital shouldn't utilize a ventilator they can't safely support. They chose the ventilator and credentialing that was right for 99 percent of their patients. But Joanna wasn't 99 percent of their patients, and they almost killed her.

Like most systems, these rules were rational, even good. They just were systemic, with no room for working with individual needs, even if ignoring those needs might be life-threatening. A system, in this situation, forces the individual into one of its squares, no matter how poorly it fits. It pushed Joanna into that square until she got sick enough to fit in there properly and almost forever.

. . .

STANDARDIZATION—THE WAY we treated Ayo, the way we treated Joanna—can be uncomfortable and often destructive; pushing people-shaped people into square boxes can be hurtful and damaging. It is also how we, as a human society, make progress. Agreeing on a standard-size metric unit is how Western civilization began to flourish; forcing our trans-Atlantic shipments into containers is how global trade became both feasible and cheap.[7] What a system can accomplish is amazing. In the medical system, there are things that never, ever get better until we make people fill out forms and checklists and follow protocols.

It's so easy to get angry at administrators, at systems, at bureaucracy, at the Kafkaesque paper pushers who won't look up from their desks. But let's talk about that clinic, the one that didn't allow for Ayo to get an MFM appointment before being referred by her prenatal care provider. Let me make a confession: I made that rule. Or perhaps, to appropriately use the language of large organizations, I was one of the administrators who developed that workflow. That is to say, I've been that bureaucrat, pushing paper (well, e-mail; unbelievable torrential tsunami-high piles of e-mail) through our medical

system. And honestly, those jobs have been some of the most satisfying ones I've ever had. Because instead of complaining about how
there were no appointments available for maternal-fetal medicine
patients, I could try to fix it. And instead of solving problems for one
patient at a time, I could solve it for a lot of people, all at once.

Here's another example. A long time ago, obstetrics called 37
weeks a "term pregnancy"—meaning that the pregnancy was completed, that the baby was ready to be out here in the world. But at
some point, the medical world started to notice that this wasn't really
always true. What we thought of as "term" pregnancies were not a
homogeneous group; not all weeks of gestation were created equal.
It turns out that babies born between 37 and 39 weeks, especially
those born without spontaneous labor, had worse outcomes. They
had more immediate problems—more NICU stays, more needs
for respiratory support. And more damningly, these babies had a
higher long-term mortality—63 percent higher.[8] (It is here that every
responsible statistician rushes in to remind us that the absolute risk
of infant mortality in the United States is extremely low, at under
6 deaths per 1,000 live births; even a 63 percent increase over that
is a low rate indeed. And yet, an avoidable 63 percent increase over
a very small baseline risk seems worth avoiding when the outcome
we're talking about is the death of a small child.)

Study after study was done, overwhelmingly showing the same
thing: choosing to deliver babies before 39 weeks, when not medically
necessary, was not a smart thing to do. For a while, nothing changed.
Individual doctors still had their ways of practice, and most of them
kept doing what they had been doing before. Eventually, national
guidelines were changed and terminology revamped. The medical
community no longer called 37-weekers "term," but expanded the

dictionary: 37 to 39 weeks was now "early-term," and 39-weekers got the more fulsome "full-term." As a result, large national organizations changed their guidelines about when delivery was recommended.

I was a young attending when these changes came out. People would read the new guidelines and nod, but faced with an uncomfortably pregnant patient or one with a family member in town, they would still schedule the cesarean as they had always done— somewhere after 37 weeks. Nothing had changed.

I tried to change things myself. I scheduled patients only after 39 weeks and tried to push back on colleagues who asked me to assist in deliveries for early-term cases. But as a lone doctor, it was an unwinnable fight; and it was unpleasant. Eventually, I gave up.

Then something changed. It wasn't explosive or exciting; it wasn't even terribly interesting. Bad medicine, it turns out, ends not with a bang, but with a whimper, crushed by the slowly grinding wheel of bureaucracy.

One day, hospital administration announced that every induction of labor and cesarean delivery prior to 39 weeks would be reviewed. If no medical reason was found in the chart, the doctors would be contacted to review the chart and explain their decision-making. If no medical reason for the early-term delivery was forthcoming, the nurse would call the physician to confirm the event and make a note of it. That was it: an X would be placed in a spreadsheet. One day, those Xs might be aggregated, or trended over time. Ultimately, there might be a graph, with bars showing a pattern of practice. But right now, there wasn't going to be any of that; just a phone call and an X in a spreadsheet.

In the hospitals I worked in, those Xs were never used in any overt way. There was no plan to change billing or compensation practice based on the rate of early-term deliveries; there was no disciplinary action involved, and there was no plan to make any of this information public or even available to colleagues. The entirety of the intervention was that attention would be paid to this issue. That's it.

And that was enough. With the light of that X from that spreadsheet shining on them, doctors began to change their practice. I saw this in the culture of my institution; doctors hated getting the call from the nurse. They hated having to explain why they had made their choice when they knew it wasn't good medicine. They hated getting their own statistics, pointing out in black and white how often they didn't follow the guidelines they knew. They hated that someone in the administrative office was paying attention.

Soon enough, they hated that more than they hated having to explain to patients why the induction couldn't just be moved a week earlier or why the cesarean wouldn't happen before Grandma's trip back to California. At my hospital, the culture changed. It became less and less usual to schedule a cesarean delivery at 38 weeks "just because"; and early-term birth rates at our hospital fell. This fall in early-term deliveries was something that became true around the country.[9]

Individuals have limited power to fix institution-wide hardened problems like these. Only systems can effectively address this kind of bad care. Bureaucracy has that power, the power of making a spreadsheet, of identifying people who are not behaving well. This small act—of paying attention to that behavior—can modify the behavior.

· · ·

SYSTEMIZATION IS ALSO powerful in that it can make things work better. Systemization can accomplish a lot without upgrading our old clunky equipment, our ancient workflow, just by standardizing the way we all do things. If we agree to work as a system, instead of as individuals, magical things can happen. My favorite example of this is the massive transfusion protocol (MTP).

One night, I attended the delivery of Lucy Fitzroy after an uncomplicated labor, following an uncomplicated pregnancy. The baby was delivered at 4:06 a.m. I was awaiting the delivery of the placenta. I was probably longing for my uncomfortable on-call room bed.

At 4:10 a.m., the placenta delivered, intact and normal.

But at 4:11 a.m., the uterus failed to contract. If the uterus does not contract, it bleeds in a way that is rarely seen outside of large motor vehicle accidents or gunshot wounds or war. When a uterus bleeds, all the blood supply that was built to grow a baby is open and bleeding out onto the floor. A friend of mine from residency, known for her gallows humor, calls this "audible bleeding"; you know that the patient is in serious trouble because you can hear the blood splashing to the floor.

That morning, we had audible bleeding. When it started, I began the easy steps: uterine massage, medications. I placed a catheter to empty Lucy's bladder and help the uterus contract. When that didn't work, when the lost blood volume was close to 1,000 milliliters, I followed our protocol and called for blood transfusion; I activated our MTP.

I called for anesthesia help and nursing help; when they came, they called for more help. They placed extra IVs; we poured in more medications. That didn't work.

I explained to Lucy and her husband what was happening; I explained that we needed to go to the operating room. I explained that I didn't know exactly what we would do in the operating room, but that we had to go, now, because her life was at risk. Lucy's husband was wide-eyed and nodded. Lucy herself was drowsy and fighting to say more than a word or two: she was going into shock from blood loss.

We took Lucy to the operating room. I called for surgical help from GYN oncology. Anesthesia put her all the way to sleep and put a tube down her throat. Blood products were pouring into Lucy's body through two IV sites but still not keeping up with the amount pouring out.

We opened Lucy's belly. Everything we touched bled: every hole our needle made, every site of contact with our cautery bled. By 5:30 a.m., we knew we had to do a hysterectomy. By 6:15 a.m., less than an hour into the surgery, the uterus was almost out, but Lucy was still bleeding. I had already done almost everything I knew how to do, and so had all the people I had called for help. I had a heavy, bilious certainty in my belly, a feeling I've only felt once or twice in my career, that this new mother was going to die.

Lucy didn't die. She didn't die, but not because I did anything extraordinary; I didn't, nor did anyone else's expertise end up being what saved her.

Lucy didn't die mostly because from the moment her hemorrhage was recognized, the MTP was activated; she had been receiving blood products, in huge volumes, without hesitation. The MTP saved her life.

Here's the old way we used to transfuse in these kinds of situations. We were slow; we were thoughtful. We sent labs and cal-

culated mathematical equations. Previously, we waited and tailored
the therapy; we waited until the need for blood became demonstra-
ble through abnormal vital signs or abnormal labs. Then we gave
just enough blood products to correct those abnormalities, and no
more. The volume of the transfusion—when to give more, what type
of blood product to give—was individualized.

Modern medicine has learned about massive transfusions from
war and from large-volume trauma in young, previously healthy people, a population more analogous to pregnant women than most of
the elderly, sick hospitalized population. Over time, we have learned
that by the time a young, healthy body is showing the stress of blood
loss, it is often too late. Once enough blood has been lost that a patient
is having trouble maintaining clotting function and vital signs, that
body has entered a spiral of poor clotting leading to more bleeding
leading to instability and death.

So we changed everything. Instead of a surgeon calling for
blood, deciding what products, and awaiting blood results, now the
whole thing is automatic. Once the MTP is activated, a cooler with
blood products in ratios proved to be most effective for most people
(1 unit red blood cells:1 unit platelets:1 unit plasma) is sent; and that
cooler is sent again and again and again until the surgical team tells
the blood bank to stop sending it. We don't give patients blood until
their labs normalize; we might not even send labs. Instead, we auto-
matically give, and give some more, without stopping to think about
it, until the bleeding has stopped. And we think it means that more
people probably live.[10]

Do you know what MTP really is? It's not new technology or a new
computer system. We've had blood transfusions for almost 300 years,
and very little about them has changed in the last 50. MTP involves all

the same surgical and anesthesiology and blood bank staff that were involved before MTP. What is different in MTP is standardization: it's that the managers of these various parts of the hospital sat down together and agreed to a protocol; they agreed to do things this way every time that they were asked, for every patient in this situation. MTP is just a list and an agreement to do the things on that list. It's bureaucratic committee work, finished up in a windowless conference room on a dull Tuesday afternoon. Without it, Lucy would be dead.

. . .

THAT BUREAUCRATIC COMMITTEE work is becoming more and more important in the United States these days. Small practices with individual doctors are a dying breed; most doctors in the United States work for a large hospital or an enormous network of large hospitals. This change—the systemization of the doctor—is also a result of the system. It is both the burden of the large system and its strength.

It's less and less feasible and financially sustainable to be a small practice and have enough resources to deal with the insanely complicated U.S. insurance industry or interface properly with multiple hospitals. It's expensive to set up an electronic medical record (EMR) and increasingly difficult to practice without one in an age when prescriptions and other necessary functions are expected to be digital. It's getting harder and harder to practice as an individual, and so fewer and fewer of us do. In fact, in my generation, we never had an assumption that we would; I graduated medical training with the idea that I would join a large group within a large department within a larger hospital, as did almost all my friends in my class.

And so, most of the doctors you know and love are not just navigators and purveyors of the modern medical system, but subjects of it as well. The doctors, also, are widgets and spreadsheet cells; few of us are individuals in this brave new world. This reality surprises most of my patients. My patients did not grow up in the age of TV shows about a kindly doctor who somehow treated a whole town;[11] they grew up with *Grey's Anatomy*. And yet, somehow they still expect their own, personal doctor; they still are crushed to find that such a creature no longer exists. My patients, but also my sophisticated cosmopolitan friends, spend weeks and months looking for the right midwife, the right doctor, and then are shocked and dismayed to find out that another doctor will likely attend their delivery, a doctor whom they may not meet until that very day.

Every day, patients ask me if I will attend their delivery. No, I have to answer, almost definitely no. No, I'm part of a large department, and I'm only on L&D the days that I'm on call, twice a month. I try to explain the positives of this: there are always doctors at the hospital devoted to being on L&D; no more providers running back and forth from hospital to clinic, exhausted and unsafe.

Nobody is happy with this explanation, ever; there's a disappointment there, and maybe more: betrayal, abandonment. I have to explain to them that although I've guided them through their choice to deliver and scheduled their cesarean delivery, they will meet the surgeon who will perform that delivery for the first time on the morning of their operation. "All of our providers are wonderful," I enthuse. "Really." None of this ever lands well. But it turns out that it isn't just the patients that are generic commodities within the medical system; it's also the doctors. And that is very hard on the patient.

But being part of the system in this way is hard for the doctor, too. It's less hard, of course; it's not our bodies being treated. But there's a hardship that comes along with being absorbed into that giant system. It's hard to work with a patient, to worry with a patient, to endure weeks and months of concern with a patient, and then not be able to be there for the delivery you worked so hard together to plan and reach. On the other side, it's demoralizing to meet that patient at 9 a.m. and convince them that yes, Dr. Karkowsky is a fully credentialed surgeon, and yes, Dr. Karkowsky is familiar with your chart, and yes, Dr. Karkowsky is basically your only option if you want the cesarean delivery today. It's hard all the way around.

The medical system is a tank; it doesn't recognize the patient's individual needs, but neither does it recognize the individual doctor's needs. We're widgets in the system, too. The system is a more powerful and effective system because of that. But being a widget wears on a person after a while, especially when that person thought they were going to be *the* doctor, but they're really only ever *a* doctor.

. . .

OF COURSE, IT wasn't always this way. For most of human history, birth was something women did at home—noninstitutionalized, unsystematized, unstandardized. It was something that women did with other women, in their own homes, often in their own beds.

Looking at the history of pregnancy and delivery care in the United States can be very revealing. The birth experience during preindustrial and industrial America is explored thoroughly in Judith Walzer Leavitt's excellent book *Brought to Bed: Childbearing in America, 1750–1950.*[12] She points out some of the tremendous advantages to births outside the hospital and outside the medical system. Caregivers were often (though not always) familiar; they were always female. There was the control over the environment that being at home allowed.

But there were, of course, serious disadvantages. Women died in birth and after birth all the time. Maternal mortality in preindustrial America was high. The heartbreaking clarity in the letters and journals of women during their pregnancies is almost painful to read. In 1890, Nannie Stillwell Jackson wrote in her diary during her pregnancy: "I told her to see after Lizzie and Sue [her first two children] if I was to die & not to let me be buried here." A pregnant Clara Clough Lenroot wrote in 1891: "It occurs to me possibly I may not live. . . . I wonder if I should die and leave a little daughter behind me, they would name her 'Clara.' I should like to have them." As Leavitt puts it, "During most of American history, an important part of women's experience of childbirth was their anticipation of dying or being permanently injured during the event."[13]

Women, naturally, wanted to change that experience. The first change was inviting physicians—male physicians—to home deliveries. And in the early twentieth century, the search for safety was one reason that birth started moving into the hospital.

There were other reasons for the move to hospitals. Often nasty campaigns by the obstetric establishment against midwives[14] had their effect. A rapidly professionalizing health care system during the Progressive Era, especially after publication of the famous Flexner Report in 1910, accelerated the shift to hospital births even more.[15] And then there was the availability of anesthesia in the hospitals. In addition, women also often didn't have the community that a home-based birth required; many of the networks that women relied on had been demolished by the mobilization and urbanization of mid-century America.[16]

However, Leavitt also says that the main reason women started to give birth in hospitals was that they wanted a safer birth. As hospitals became reputedly safer in general—as germ theory began to be accepted and aseptic techniques widespread through medical institutions—upper- and middle-class women, followed shortly by everyone else, fought to deliver within medical institutions. By 1940, 55 percent of America's births were in-hospital births; by 1950, it was almost 90 percent; and by 1960, outside of some isolated rural areas, it was almost unheard of for an American woman to deliver her baby at home.[17]

In those early years of hospital births, the safety advantages were more of reputation than reality. The medical system had made promises it wasn't keeping: maternal mortality rates were initially higher within hospitals; urban rates of postpartum infection increased particularly in those years of the 1920s, an indication that hospitals may have increased maternity-related infections for women.[18]

At that point, women could have fled the hospitals and returned to home birth, but that's not what happened, at least not then. Births increased at the hospitals; labor and delivery became solidly within the territory of medical institutions, and the medical system started to take responsibility and investigate its own failures within its care of childbirth.

By the early 1930s, it was common for doctors to blame themselves for preventable deaths of postpartum women.[19] Countless individual physicians and multiple organizations went on record in that decade, demonstrating that physicians and hospitals exacerbated the dangers to pregnant women, including a landmark New York Academy of Medicine report proclaiming that over half of maternal deaths were the fault of physicians themselves and that hospitals exacerbated the dangers of childbirth.[20]

Aided by these revelations and by improved record-keeping

about preventable deaths, the leading hospitals of the time did what large systems do: they moved toward regulation and standardization of hospital obstetrics. They decreased the overuse and misuse of operative procedures and of sedating drugs. By the 1940s and 1950s, hospital regulation increased and led, in part, to the success seen in reducing infections and hemorrhages, two of the largest contributors to maternal mortality. By the mid-twentieth century, childbirth was safer than it had ever been in the United States.[21]

When women started going to hospitals to deliver their babies in the early twentieth century, birth in a large institution wasn't less dangerous. But women wanted it to be; they needed it to be. In pursuit of a safe delivery, those women advocated to be included within the formal institutions of the medical system. Faced with these patients, the medical system used the tools it did have: systemization, standardization, bureaucratization. Eventually, those women did get the safer hospital delivery that they had sought.

That's not the end of the story: in the 1950s, women became increasingly unhappy with in-hospital deliveries, with the loss of control over their experience and their bodies that a hospital birth began to represent. During the mid-twentieth century and onward, women began to advocate to change those hospital routines so that they could have safe deliveries that still respected their agency and dignity, to integrate the warmth and intimacy of home delivery rooms with the safety and hygiene they had come to expect from hospital care.[22] Changes were made; the famous actress Julie Harris, for example, fought an extremely public battle in the 1950s to have her husband in the delivery room with her, and now that kind of support from a partner during childbirth is both expected and routine.

More recently, women have demanded even more changes in

the childbirth system. However, instead of advocating for change within the hospital system, women are now leaving it. In the United States, planned home births have been rising primarily among higher-income women, the same socioeconomic group that led the march of childbirth into the hospital over 100 years ago. There are many reasons for this move, including an increasing mistrust of science and expertise within our culture.[23] But many of those women are searching for a way out of the systematization, standardization, and bureaucratization that the modern medical system represents.

It's an understandably appealing option for some people: the comfort and individualization of being outside the medical institution, assuming the safety of a hospital birth is preserved. But can you assume that safety? This question, it turns out, is a hard one to answer. The data on the safety of home deliveries are complicated and mixed, their studies generally hard to conduct. For one thing, it's always hard to study people who move themselves outside the system. For another, it's also hard to separate the patient who had planned a home birth from the one who unintentionally delivered in the hospital parking lot on the way to the labor floor.

The best studies of planned home birth thus far have found a decrease in interventions such as operative vaginal delivery, cesarean delivery, and episiotomy, although these lower numbers would be expected for the low-risk women that are generally found pursuing a home birth. Some studies have found a marked increase in neonatal mortality: approximately triple that of a hospital birth, although other studies dispute this finding.[24]

It's important to note that almost all rigorous controlled studies of planned home birth generally study home births where care is provided by highly educated and certified midwives who are well integrated into the health care system and where extremely strict criteria include only the lowest-risk women for a planned home birth.[25] In particular, it's important to realize that studies looking at planned home birth with more permissive criteria for including patients do demonstrate a markedly higher neonatal mortality rate.[26]

That's an important distinction, because in the United States, planned home birth can represent a whole spectrum of experiences with a whole spectrum of providers. In many states, and for many women, home birth is, by design and usually by intention, outside of the medical system. (In some states, planned home birth is also something that occurs outside the law.[27]) Depending on the state and the preferences of the woman in question, planned home birth in the United States is often outside of any systematizing, standardizing impulses.

Let's take credentialing and education as an example. In many states, home births are almost never attended by a doctor and only a minority of the time by a highly educated and regulated professional with a certified nurse midwife (CNM) or certified midwife (CM) credential.[28] This means that birth attendants for home births may be CNM/CMs; but they also may hold a less regulated certification, such as certified professional midwife (CPM). There are about 30 states where CPMs are licensed and regulated.[29] But even within the group of CPMs who are credentialed, wide variations in educational requirements and state regulatory conditions exist.[30]

In states where the CPM credential is not available, the providers who attend home birth are not necessarily holders of these or any particular degree or credential. They may be; it's just that in those states, these birth attendants exist outside of regulatory practice.[31]

Birth attendants in unregulated states may have a variety

of credentialing or none, a variety of experiential knowledge or not enough. They may practice science-based or evidence-based therapies—or they may not. They may not be able to get the medications I use every day to stop postpartum bleeding, because those require a prescription (something one needs to be within the system to acquire). Many of these birth attendants may know more than I ever will about normal birth; but some of them may not know nearly enough about identifying and managing complications. In those states, nobody is checking, because validating credentials is something that happens within a system.

And what happens when everything isn't absolutely fine? Transfer from a planned home birth to a hospital birth is not infrequent. Somewhere between 10 and 40 percent of planned home-birth patients are transferred to a hospital after the onset of labor.[32] Being outside the system means that getting inside the system when you need to can be very difficult. In many of those arrangements, there's no relationship with a hospital or a doctor; there are no agreed-upon criteria for transferring care to the hospital and no workflow to accomplish this quickly. Anyone who works in labor and delivery is acutely aware of how quickly things can change.

I work in a hospital, so of course the only home births I've seen have been the ones with problems, the ones that need transfer, the ones that fail. That's not fair, of course; I won't ever see all the ones that go well. Despite my very particular experiences, I am aware that the vast majority of planned home births go well. Many of them go better than they would have within my system, with all my resources. But I am, by definition of my training and my experience, a biased observer.

The planned home births that I do see—the transfers, the failures—exhibit particularly well what happens when someone outside the system urgently needs to cross the chasm between outside the system and inside the system and how much that chasm can cost.

One case I particularly remember was a woman with two prior cesareans who had desperately wanted a vaginal delivery. Her labor was something that all obstetric guidelines at the time prohibited because her uterine rupture rate (see Chapter 6) was unacceptably high according to all the obstetric rule-making bodies. Her desire and plan for a labor was rejected by multiple hospitals near her home in the southwestern United States. In these days before the idea of CPM certification existed, she ended up seeking out a woman who was famous in these circles of women who wanted to avoid the hospital, someone without formal nursing or medical background who attended births. This birth attendant pledged to keep this patient out of the hospital. The patient moved her family to our city to be near this birth attendant and await labor.

On the day this patient went into labor, after some long hours of contractions, the birth attendant emergently brought the patient to the hospital. I won't ever know what finally pushed her to this act. I remember that the patient had been 6 centimeters for several hours with thick meconium. Were there dips in the fetal heart rate? I don't know if the birth attendant was monitoring the fetal heart rate intermittently or at all. The patient may also have had a fever. All I remember was the lack of clarity, the muzziness of the transfer: there were no records, none of that data that we were used to accessing to care for patients. Nobody had called an ambulance; the patient was driven by the birth attendant in a regular car, flashing hazard lights the whole way through a crowded highway. I don't remember much about the patient herself—I was very junior at the time—but I do remember that as soon as she was put on the fetal heart rate monitor, what they saw was concerning enough that she was whisked away to the operating room. I remember that the case was delayed because putting an IV in a dehydrated laboring patient is tough. And I remember that the senior resident said that the surgery was a difficult one, as would be the case after two prior operations on the same organs, and that this delayed delivery even more. I remember in the days after this delivery that there was a lot of murmuring about the baby, first about the low Apgar scores and later about EEGs and concern for abnormal brain activity.

I don't know how that story ended; I don't know how that baby is doing today. The only thing I remember is that the day after that surgery, morning rounds on L&D were buzzing with anger: There was anger that the patient had been managed so badly, that the decision to transfer wasn't made hours or days or months earlier. This was a patient who never should have been in labor outside the hospital, said all the young doctors. There was anger on behalf of the baby who wasn't doing well, who we could have saved, and anger on the part of the patient, who still seemed dazed by all that had happened, stunned that her faith—in her body, in her birth attendant—had not been realized.

And, I think, there was also anger from the doctors that participating in this kind of traumatic case was traumatic to us, too. The management of this birth attendant put us all in a difficult situation; now we were all participants in a disaster not of our own making or of our own choosing. Someone rejected our system and all the resources that came with it, all our work and education and expertise, until the moment they came in and demanded every single one of those things urgently. They demanded all of our gifts exactly when those gifts would not and could not be enough, exactly when we would fail them.

During those morning rounds, the head of L&D, a venerable gray-haired professor, made a point of standing up. He said something like this: "What you need to know is that I invited the care provider in this case, the birth attendant, to be in the OR with us. I asked her opinion after the case. I will call her today, as well, to discuss the patient. I am not doing any of this because I agree with how she practices. I don't think she knows obstetrics better than me, better than us. I don't agree with how she manages her patients in general, and I'm upset about this patient in particular. But I do know this: if I include her in the patient's care; if I don't isolate her from the patient; if I show her that I respect her judgment, maybe next time she will not hesitate for so long to bring the patient to us. That's what I want you to learn from this case."

There was a chasm between the world of that birth attendant and our hospital world, a gap that took too long for this patient to cross when she needed it. In the aftermath, the head of L&D was trying to bridge that chasm. He knew that there were other patients out there making these choices, and he wanted what was best for these patients who would continue to leave the medical system and pursue birth in a world that he had no other connection or relationship to. I remember thinking back then that this was a virtuous and correct course of action; I remember being proud of my institution for its nobility.

I didn't think, back then, in that buzzing conference room, of the poverty of the options that the patient had to choose from early in her pregnancy. I didn't think, back then, that because of the way systems worked for her, the only choices she had felt to her like terrible ones. She was required to either agree to a major surgery she didn't want or leave the system.

It hadn't occurred to me that it wasn't only the birth attendant or the patient who had made choices leading to this situation, who had created this damage, but that we, the institutions—the hospital in the Southwest, the hospital in the Northeast, the professional association that had written those VBAC guidelines—had made some of those choices as well. Our wealthy systems, so immersed in our richness of resources and legitimacy that we didn't even see them, had kept that wealth to ourselves. Could we have figured out a way to allow that patient to try labor inside our institution after counseling her about the risk? Could we have created a way for her to have agency over her body while staying within our walls? Was there a way to allow her access to our wealth while letting her reject our advice?

Now, looking back, I think there has to be a better way. Why does this stark binary—either out of the system or wholly in it—exist? Is there a middle path?

In the Netherlands, home birth is an entirely different entity. Planned home birth is a relatively common option—20 percent of women in the Netherlands have one. But this option, for them, isn't outside the medical system. For this country, planned home birth is an integrated part of medical care. Strict guidelines exist for which patients are eligible for planned home birth; midwives are credentialed; protocols exist for both routine maternal transfer and obstetric emergencies.

Women labor and mostly deliver at home; but they do so within the advantages of a system, even if they're not within the walls of its institution. They deliver with protocols and with preexisting relationships: with a registered midwife in their home and a doctor who is responsive and responsible at the hospital, if need be. They can be individuals but still have access to safety algorithms and transfer protocols. They can be outside and inside the system at the same time.

· · ·

THERE ARE WAYS, then, to cross the divide. Hopefully, one day there will be more creative ways to prioritize a patient's (and maybe even a doctor's) personal and wholly singular experience while reaping the gains that can be made by an enormous system.

As for me, today, I'm writing this at the side of my daughter's hospital bed. She is 3 years old. She went to sleep healthy but with a runny nose. At 2 a.m. I heard her gasping, choking, hungry for air; she was wide-eyed, without enough breath to cry. I was scared, confused, and barely awake. I threw pants on, put her on my hip and ran out of the apartment; within 10 minutes, we were at a major hospital. I ran into the emergency department lobby, with no medical cool about me, shouting, "Shortness of breath, shortness of breath!" The secretary, hearing her gasps, waved us past: Go already! Go to the doctors! We bypassed the medical paperwork and ran into the patient area, where we were swarmed by several nurses and a doctor; within 5 minutes, my daughter was assessed and treatment begun; within 10 minutes, she was able to cry.

And yet, that moment didn't last; the medical system requires its due. As soon as my daughter was out of acute distress, the doctors asked me to step back outside to the desk. "It's hard for us to get meds out for her until you register her within the system," they said. "It'll just take a few minutes." I didn't want to leave her, even for a moment—she's still so little—but the system required it.

I squeezed her hand and ran back out to that front desk, digging through my backpack for her insurance card, waving it in front of that same secretary, who clicked through her screens with agonizing slowness.

This afternoon, almost 24 hours later, what my toddler is still talking about, over and over again, is those few minutes alone:

"I didn't like that you left me, Mama. Why you leave me, Mama?"

"I'm sorry; I didn't like it either, sweetheart. But I had to."

We have this conversation twice, then five times, then ten.

Did I have to leave her, though? Couldn't a pediatric emergency room system, presumably dealing with similar situations every day, come up with a better way to register young patients? But those were the terms of the system, and I was in no position to bargain.

Today, also, my toddler is breathing beautifully. She is breathing so beautifully that we are ready to go home, have been ready for hours now. We are awaiting routine paperwork, paperwork that I don't need, forms that will change absolutely nothing, but which the system requires and which some medical trainee is working on. My daughter has spent those hours systematically dismembering the bathroom toilet paper dispenser, gorging on cartoons, and repeatedly asking me, "Why you leave me, Mama?" before finally falling asleep.

She is sleeping quietly, though with dark circles under her eyes. I've turned off the lights. The pediatric resident walks by and assures me that the paperwork will be done in the next hour; 2 hours, max. I sit here, uncomfortably wedged into the bed next to my baby, typing in the dark illuminated by numbers from her oxygen monitor. I'm watching her breathe and am breathing next to her, for 1 hour, and then 2, and now heading into a third.

In these moments, waiting for the system to finish its slow col-
lation of her illness and the indexing of her particular precious
small body, all of those stupidities of the medical system—the "Why
you leave me, Mama?," the paperwork, the delays—are trivial; they
are nothing to me. In the dim twilight of this room, with my child
inhaling and exhaling into the hollow of my left elbow, most of what
I feel is deep and profound thankfulness for that medical system. I
could weep right now with the weight of my gratitude for the system
we ran into at 2 o'clock in the morning, without air; and that we will
leave, breathing easily, whenever that paperwork is done.

POSTPARTUM AND BEYOND

10.

Maternal Mortality and Racial Disparities in Health Care

Implicit, Complicit

Sometimes, even those of us who work here forget that women can die.

Long ago, I was leading a day of communication skills training for the residents. We chose as our simulated scenario the diagnosis of stillbirth (see Chapter 7).

"Wow," said one of my colleagues. "You're not going easy on them, are you? You're just starting with the nuclear situation."

What I said out loud was, "Believe it or not, they requested this topic."

But what I said in my head was, "Stillbirth is not the nuclear situation. The nuclear situation is when a woman dies. Our apocalyptic scenario is not fetal mortality; it's maternal mortality. And you know that."

Maternal mortality is, thankfully, rare. It happens far less often than fetal mortality. Sometimes it's infrequent enough that we can pretend it doesn't happen at all. But it does happen: women die during and after pregnancy much too often. More worrisome, women are dying during and after pregnancy more than they were a decade ago. Somehow, despite our best efforts, we are getting worse at this, not better.[1]

In terms of absolute raw numbers, the risk of dying from childbirth in the United States is low: 23.8 deaths per 100,000 births. But this rate is drawing more and more attention because it's one of the highest in the world for a high-income country. That is, we spend a lot of money on health care—more per capita than almost any other country in the world[2]—and women are dying more than ever. And worse, this growing tragedy is a shamefully biased one: black women are dying more than white women. We're doing something wrong.

That number, 23.8 per 100,000, means that those of us in this line of work won't see a maternal death for a year, or two, or even five. Like that colleague at my simulation training, we can then forget what it means: how terrible it is; that it can happen at all. But when it does happen, it is a nuclear bomb: it lays waste to everything and everyone nearby for years after.

.   .   .

EVEN IN A hospital, where death and blood are routine, a maternal death is something big and horrible. It is a catastrophe, and it is experienced and treated as such.

What I'm going to describe as the provider experience in this situation is, of course, nothing compared with the trauma that the family undergoes. But even so, I remember every single maternal death that I have ever been near, even if I didn't meet most of these women or participate in their care. When I say I was near these deaths, what

I mean is that these women died at an institution while I worked there. And even if I didn't make any of the decisions related to their care or even meet them, I remember the grief and tragedy pervading the hallways; I remember the quiet discussions, the tears, and the shock for days after, then months after, even years after.

The first maternal mortality I encountered occurred when I had just started a rotation on L&D at the very beginning of my training. I was new to the hospital, new to L&D, and disoriented most of the time. I heard rumors in the hallway, noticed white-faced medical students still shaking from what had happened. I found one colleague slumped over in the stairwell, weeping.

Here is the version that I heard: The patient, whom I'll call Kayla, had been in labor, at term. She had been 8 centimeters for a long time and never progressed further. After some time, she was taken to the operating room for cesarean delivery. The cesarean was, reportedly, uncomplicated.

After the cesarean, Kayla's blood pressure was low. The nurse called the anesthesia resident, who assumed that her low blood pressure was a side effect of her anesthesia, yet to wear off. That resident gave Kayla a medication to increase her blood pressure. It worked, but just for 15 minutes or so, and then Kayla's blood pressure fell again. The anesthesia resident and the nurse realized at this point that something else was very, very wrong. They called for the obstetrics team and sent off blood work, and it became clear that Kayla was bleeding internally. She was taken to the operating room; transfusions were started. I don't know at what point it was too late, but at some point, it was too late. Kayla died in the operating room.

I was too junior and too peripheral to the department to be truly involved in discussions. There was presumably a morbidity and mortality conference about Kayla's death, though I don't think I attended it. What I remember is more subtle: harrowed looks, whispered conversations in the hallway, and a lot of silence. I saw attending physicians—so senior to me, so forbidding during morning rounds—looking exhausted and scared, sometimes leaning against each other. I half-heard about meetings and investigations and perhaps a physician placed under suspension. Months later, postcesarean recovery protocols were reviewed and revamped.

To me, the process seemed never-ending and unclear: it was at times a search for blame and at times a search for repentance. And when those endeavors were exhausted, the grief that remained was channeled into what medical institutions do best (see Chapter 9): trying to review, rebuild, and systematize so we never, ever do this to anyone ever again. But of course it wasn't enough. Maternal mortality still existed, and it happened again, to someone else somewhere else.

. . .

HERE'S THE STORY of another maternal death, one that happened slightly later in my training. I'm going to call her Violet, although, like Kayla, I never met her and never learned her real name. I was working on labor and delivery (L&D) at the time of this story, but Violet never made it to labor and delivery.

Weeks before the event, Violet's water had broken, sometime in the middle of her second trimester. She was given the same counseling that we offered to everyone in that situation: that prognosis was poor, that reaching viability at 23 or 24 weeks was unlikely, and that even if she made it that far, developing without amniotic fluid was known to cause major problems for the fetus. The chance for a live baby from this pregnancy was extremely low and for a healthy baby even lower. And continuing the pregnancy came with risks for her—infection, bleeding. I don't know if they mentioned death; death is a rare complication of continuing pregnancy with ruptured membranes, but death is a rare complication of almost everything.

As standard care dictates, Violet was offered an induction of labor or a dilation and evacuation (D&E)—both ways to terminate her pregnancy—as the safest course of action. Violet didn't want any of this, and she left the hospital, presumably signing out against medical advice (see Chapter 8). I don't know if she had appointments in a clinic or if she just left and spent weeks at home. I heard, distantly, that she was angry, dissatisfied with the care offered to her and with all of the terrible options laid before her.

I was early in my training during Violet's story. I had never dealt with this kind of situation, of breaking water at 18 weeks. Since then, I have seen similar situations countless times. Most women in this situation either go into labor or get an infection. Of those who don't, most accept an induction of labor as the safest option. But I still have seen women make Violet's choice—to continue the pregnancy—many times. Most of the time, nothing good happens but nothing terribly dangerous happens. Women who make this choice usually go into labor or get a fever and come back in; if that happens, usually they need to be given antibiotics and to be delivered. And rarely, rarely, they get to or past viability; even more rarely, there's a live baby at the end. It's almost always a tragic situation, but it's rarely life-threatening to the patient making this choice.

But back then, I was new; I had never seen the management of a second-trimester rupture of membranes or heard the counseling. I had never seen a patient accept or reject our care. Back then, all I heard was a hubbub late one afternoon, when all the available doctors left L&D to run to the emergency room, leaving me with just one attending upstairs. Later I heard the summary: Violet had returned after some period of time at home, either days or weeks. She appeared in the emergency room, feverish, sick, and in shock. It was immediately clear that Violet's uterus and pregnancy had become infected. Antibiotics were started. Plans were immediately initiated: Induction of labor in the ICU? Evacuation of the uterus down in the operating room if she was stable enough?

None of it mattered because by the time Violet came in, she was too sick. Within minutes of coming in to the hospital, her blood pressure dropped, and then her heart stopped beating. I assume that the team resuscitated her and performed a code for hours; she was a young healthy woman, and sometimes we can get them back. But we didn't get Violet back. Violet died that night.

. . .

LET'S TAKE A step back from Kayla and Violet for a moment. If we want to really understand maternal mortality, we need to look at it on a larger scale—by city or state or country or the world. Worldwide, the obstetric causes of maternal mortality are those associated with low-income countries: hemorrhage; hypertensive diseases of pregnancy such as preeclampsia and eclampsia; unsafe abortion; infections; obstructed labor. Many of these causes are things that those of us in high-income countries think we've extinguished—or at least we know how to deal with them. We have blood banks and clean operating rooms and medications to lower blood pressure. We are so lucky; we are so rich. Our maternal mortality rate is too high, we think, but we know how to fix this. We haven't fixed it yet; but we know how. We just need to get around to it.

The picture in the United States is actually more complicated. When we look at obstetric causes of maternal mortality, we see limited change over time; since 2006, for example, there has been a reduction in deaths from hemorrhage, hypertensive disorders of pregnancy, and anesthesia complications, with an increase in deaths from cardiovascular disease and other medical conditions.[3] That is, some of these deaths are more connected to the general health of the women who enter pregnancy, women who are often older and less healthy, and with less access to health care, than in prior times.

But really, the numbers sliced this way aren't the whole story. What's more informative is to look at the deaths of mothers by race and ethnicity. When we do this, we see the shameful truth: black women are dying in the United States more than anyone else and more than ever.

.   .   .

ACCORDING TO THE CDC Pregnancy Mortality Surveillance System, from 2011 to 2014, pregnancy-related mortality rates for black women were 3.2 times that for white women.[4] When factoring in variables that protect against maternal mortality—higher education, higher socioeconomic status, enrolling in prenatal care—those advantages do not protect black women; they reduce the risk of death, but not enough to make it anywhere near equal to risk for white women.[5] This means that a black woman entering pregnancy is more likely to die. It also means that nothing else about her influences her risk of death in pregnancy in the United States as much as the color of her skin.

As a doctor—as part of that medical system—learning this is something that occurs in stages that are similar to grief. First, disbelief: it can't possibly be true; I try so hard; everyone I know tries so hard; it can't be true. Then acceptance: it is true; I see from the statistics that it is true. And following immediately, a deep well of shame, almost existential in its depth. How can this be the result of the work we do? How can we continue this work when this work is going so terribly wrong?

Then, later, the indisputable realization that it's worse than that. It's not the work that creates this problem; and it's not "them," a group of nameless evil doctors somewhere. It's us. And, on the days when I have the strength to be completely honest, it's me.

· · ·

KAYLA, WHO DIED postoperatively, was black. When she complained of pain, she was given more pain medicines, because of course she had pain—she had just undergone major surgery—so they soothed her and medicated her. Did they pay as much attention as they should have to her increasing need for pain medication?

Kayla was also obese; obese patients are another group that receive suboptimal care.[6] In this case, when Kayla's blood pressure was low, the clinicians' first response was probably skepticism. Sometimes these blood pressure cuffs give funny numbers when used on obese women. Usually, their numbers are much too high, but when Kayla's number was much too low, the doubt already existed. So the team spent some time—maybe more time than they should have—getting a larger cuff and taking and retaking her blood pressure, until they finally believed that the low number was real.

In that lost time, a life was lost. Would this have happened if she had been slender? Would it have happened if she had been white?

I know the answer and so do you. The answer is "maybe." And I'm not sure how to go to work with that answer or how to live with it.

. . .

HOW COULD THIS happen? How could Kayla die? But also, how can we have a system where someone with Kayla's skin color walks into the hospital with a risk of death three to four times that of a white woman? And what part of that three to four times higher risk is the doctor's fault? What part is mine?

There is a growing body of literature investigating racial discrepancies in obstetric care. And this attention is appropriate, because it's a national emergency. In general, the beginning of any understanding of health care disparities starts by dividing the causes into three main levels: patient, provider, and system.[7] Now that the medical establishment is beginning to understand the scope and depth of this issue, there's a lot of work on all three levels.[8] But in order for me to go to work tomorrow, I want to try to understand how much of this problem is me.

The current understanding of how physician bias contributes to this discrepant care has little to do with overt racism. When surveyed, physicians in general are more likely than the general population to abhor racist attitudes or any suggestion of prejudicial principles.[9]

But the differential outcomes by race are there. So where is physician racism hiding? As the landmark 2003 Institute of Medicine report on the topic asked:

> How then, could a well-meaning group of healthcare professionals, working in their usual circumstances with diverse populations of patients, create a pattern of care that appears (on the now substantial weight of available scientific evidence) to be

discriminatory? In other words, is it possible for physicians and
other healthcare professionals to act in a racially biased manner
without knowing it?[10]

The answer is yes. There are many studies looking at how race changes our well-intentioned practice. For example, a 1999 study looked at physician recommendations for simulated patients with chest pain, where the actor-patients varied only in race, gender, and exercise habits. This study found that physicians were 40 percent less likely to recommend treatment for a heart attack, a cardiac catheterization, for women and African-Americans than for white men.[11]

This study—and many others in many other fields of medicine—demonstrates implicit bias, the immediate beliefs and attitudes that we are unable or unwilling to express.[12] (For a fuller understanding and a truly eye-opening experience, head to the Project Implicit website and take at least one of the tests provided.)

Implicit bias is made up of the small, involuntary reactions we all have to other people. We all feel warmth toward someone who speaks the same language as us or who looks like our grandma. That's normal; it's part of being human and part of processing the world. But that also means that we have certain feelings or predisposed images or thoughts toward people who have a certain skin color or a certain religion or a certain country of origin. These responses aren't voluntary, but they also aren't fair or just. To pretend otherwise is to render ourselves unable to acknowledge, much less fix, the problem.

These reactions, positive toward some people and negative toward others, constitute the implicit bias that we all exhibit, including doctors. And because white males make up a disproportionately large percentage of U.S. doctors (currently, 75 percent),[13] that's the group of clinicians that most patients, whatever their racial background, are interacting with. In contrast, African-American doctors make up only 4 percent of U.S. doctors, even though black people make up 14 percent of the U.S. population.[14] (Thankfully, this is changing dramatically; when we look at young doctors and medical students, we see more people of color and more women; the future of medicine will look different, though it will take decades.[15])

These implicit preferences are indeed small; they may not meaningfully influence any particular daily interaction; they may not be obvious in a conversation between coworkers or in every particular employment offer or in the medication choice for an individual patient. That's why they're so easy to ignore.

But like many other small but persistent forces, implicit bias is strong in aggregate. It acts on populations over time, pushing averages a particular way. As part of any society, those little biases multiply. Implicit bias is the current scientific understanding of this apparent contradiction: nobody thinks they're racist, but the care manifestly is. Studies show that white job applicants get about 50 percent more callbacks than black applicants with the same resume;[16] that college professors are more likely to schedule a meeting with a student who signs his e-mail Brad rather than Lamar;[17] and that in health care, black patients are prescribed less pain medication and fewer cardiac catheterizations. And black mothers die more often during and after pregnancy.

. . .

CHRISTINA ALEXANDER WAS a black woman, a lawyer, married. She came in at 32 weeks for an evaluation for bleeding; she told the nurse she had seen several clots in the toilet, some as large as her fist.

She was elegant and beautifully dressed; she had rushed to us directly from her law office; she was the kind of woman who had not compromised on the height of her high heels, despite entering her third trimester of pregnancy. Christina's husband met her in our triage bay, rumpled from his day of teaching school and his dash to the hospital.

The nurse didn't think the spotting Christina showed her was impressive, despite Christina's description from earlier in the day. When she told the triage doctor about Christina, she was dismissive in her description of the bleeding. The triage doctor went to see Christina; he heard her story; he also assumed that Christina's descriptions were exaggerated. That doctor performed an examination, which was unremarkable; Christina wasn't actively bleeding by this point. He reassured Christina and discharged her home.

Nobody sent labs on Christina. Nobody considered offering her steroid injections, which can reduce a lot of serious complications a baby can experience from premature birth. These injections are our first recommendation if there's any clinical suspicion that something serious might be going on, something that might lead to the need to deliver her pregnancy early. Nobody recommended that she be admitted for 24-hour observation. Because if you ignored what Christina was saying about her bleeding—if you interpreted it as "spotting" and nothing more—then none of that was necessary.

Christina returned, hemorrhaging, less than 12 hours later. She was rushed to the operating room. She underwent an emergency cesarean delivery for a very premature baby.

Christina didn't die, and despite a rough road in the NICU, neither did her baby. But if someone had taken her report of bleeding more seriously at that triage visit, her care would have been different in a lot of important ways. If that had all happened, when

Christina started bleeding again, she would have been with us, in the hospital; she would have had an IV in; and her baby would have received the benefits of those steroids. None of that happened, even though Christina was married, even though she was an educated professional.

This wasn't Jim Crow racism: Christina wasn't turned away; everyone she encountered was warm, even kind. It would be impossible to prove conclusively that Christina's own report of what she saw was dismissed because she was black. But somehow, she got labeled as a less-than-reliable witness; nobody took her report quite seriously. That small perception changed her care, for her and for her premature baby. That's what implicit bias does in a room.

. . .

Long ago, I was part of the team taking care of a patient named Janina Hodges. She was black and young, perhaps 19. She was pregnant with twins when her water broke at 20 weeks. She was very, very sad and very, very scared.

When Janina came into the hospital, she was alone. She was counseled by our attending, a prominent white female physician. This doctor sat down with Janina and told her honestly about the poor prognosis, the risks, and the high likelihood that neither of her twins would make it. The doctor was clear, though her manner wasn't terribly warm. But she was patient and took her time. She recommended, as is standard in these cases, an induction of labor. She was careful not to push Janina.

Janina was overwhelmed and asked for time to think. She wanted to wait until her boyfriend, Aaron, arrived. The attending told her that of course she could wait, but she also told Janina that her white blood count was a bit elevated; we were worried about an impending infection. She repeated to Janina that a quick decision was important. Janina leaned back in her bed and asked us to turn out the light so she could rest and think, and I think so that we wouldn't see her crying.

An hour later, I returned to the room. I had misoprostol, the medication to start the induction of labor, in my pocket. I thought Janina would agree that we could place it now; she had seemed scared when the attending had mentioned infection and our concern for any additional delay.

But in that hour, Aaron had joined her in the room. He was also young, also black. He was tall and thin and had folded himself up on the windowsill, his knees almost up to his ears; in the semidarkness, it was impossible to see his face.

When I entered the room, he came down off the windowsill and sat in a chair, leaning forward, tense and eager. That's when I saw his face: rigid, tight, eyebrows bunching in the middle. He started talking, and it became clear that he wasn't just tense; he was angry. He was furious with all of this; with all of us. With me.

Aaron started off by asking, and then almost yelling, "Why are you pushing her to have a labor? Why can't we wait and see if it will be okay?" His questions became more complex, more pointed: "Why are you pushing to kill my babies? Why can't you at least save the twin whose water didn't break?"

And later, louder: "Why don't you value my babies? Why don't you value my family?" with a push forward of his arms, an explosive extension of his hands that meant the individual Dr. Karkowsky "you," but also the collective "you," the hospital "you," the world "you."

I remember standing there, my hand creasing the envelope of misoprostol, turning it over and over in the pocket of my still-new white coat. I didn't bring the envelope out; I didn't mention it. I looked over at Janina, waiting for her to tell me what she wanted to do; legally, this was her body and her decision alone. Janina was still lying back on her pillow with her eyes closed, and she shook her head when I talked to her; she didn't want to talk to me either.

I was a smart intern. I knew how to place misoprostol, and I knew all its side effects and its pharmacological properties. But I knew nothing about what to do during this situation. So I turned around and left.

. . .

NOBODY IN THAT room mentioned race. Nobody mentioned that the attending was white, and the nurse was white, and I was white, and the patient was black, and the boyfriend was black, and the fetuses would be black. But I could understand what Aaron meant, even when he didn't say it. Aaron had brought a lifetime of hard lessons in American racism into that room. He had a deep and well-earned suspicion that a majority-white medical establishment would never value his unborn children enough.

Nobody in that room mentioned a lot of other things: tragedy, grief, mourning; wishes, hopes, dreams, nightmares. Nobody mentioned the human experience that Janina and Aaron were going through.

That room, when I turned around and left, was full of so much anger, spoken and unspoken. I left because I didn't know then how to deal with it.

Looking back, I think that what Aaron was reacting to was, at least in part, the pressure, the haste, an edge of "let's get this over with" that was in all of our recommendations. His experience in the United States led him to believe that that edge was there because of their race, their youth, and their poverty. He felt that all these biases were affecting the care and counseling they were receiving.

And I think that Aaron was right; implicit biases were in that room, as they are in every room. I think that the counseling would have been different, perhaps warmer or kinder, if Janina and Aaron had been 25, or married, or white. Perhaps the clinical care would have been different; or if it was the same, perhaps it would have been less painful. Perhaps my attending would have been warmer; perhaps I would have been.

Aaron was right. There was bias in Janina's room. But those implicit biases were not the only unspoken presence there. The other presence in the room, the ghost that was unacknowledged but heavy and visible only to the medical staff, was Violet.

Violet had died at our institution only a few months prior. The attending, the nurse, and I never mentioned Violet's death to Aaron or Janina; we never mentioned maternal death at all. It is, after all, a rare outcome, one so dramatic that even mentioning it feels violent. We didn't even mention it to each other.

Aaron was right: there was an urgency to our counseling, a shadow. Part of that shadow was the racial and ethnic and socioeconomic bias that did affect his and Janina's care and their lives up to that point and that was present now. But part of that shadow was Violet's ghost. It was the anxiety of all these providers: watching a story so similar to Violet's unfold and wanting, so desperately, to give it a different ending.

. . .

WHEN I LEFT, unequipped to deal with the anger in that room, I knew I had to get someone older and smarter than me. I ended up with my chief resident, another white woman, who explained the situation again to Janina and Aaron. She repeated the same boilerplate counseling as the attending: poor prognosis, elevated white blood cells, significant risk of infection, pregnancy termination recommended. Nothing she said changed the situation in the room: Aaron, glowering from a chair; Janina lying back in her bed. The anger was still there, and so was the ghost.

But at the end of this second conversation, my chief resident pushed. She asked Janina to make a decision. "I need an answer soon," she said. Janina could start her induction now; if she wanted to wait or didn't want an induction, we'd move her off the labor floor to a less intensively monitored bed. We needed the bed here for laboring or sick patients.

Janina cleared her throat and consented to the medication; she then lay back, closed her eyes, and didn't speak again. Aaron, tense and still angry, didn't say anything. My chief resident left the room, leaving me with the nurse and with Janina and Aaron. I took out my little creased envelope of misoprostol, put on a glove, and placed the tiny pills near Janina's cervix.

An hour later, Janina spiked a very high fever, shaking uncontrollably. Her pulse shot up, though her blood pressure stayed stable. We started antibiotics; we started talking quietly about other ways to evacuate Janina's uterus in case she started to get sicker. None of them ended up being necessary: Janina delivered quickly later that evening.

There was concern for retained placenta, a common issue in very preterm births and in twin births; but both placentas delivered easily. There was worry for bleeding because of the multiple pregnancy and the infection; but in the end, Janina bled, but not very much.

Janina and Aaron's babies were dead before they were born. Like all babies born that early, they didn't have black skin or white skin; they were still developing their skin. They were waxy and bruised, and the skin they had was translucent, no real color at all.

A few hours after her delivery, Janina's pulse started to normalize. By the morning, she had no fever, and we transferred her to the gynecology floor. By the following afternoon, she was walking around. She was wearing her own clothes and eating regular food and ready to go home.

· · ·

I'M BETTER AT this kind of situation than I was. But none of the answers I have are complete ones, and none of them are easy.

When I look back at Janina and Aaron's care, I now have the advantage of the ongoing research in this field and ongoing training in cultural competency. According to that work, perhaps the best answer would have been to have had a different doctor come speak to them, ideally a black doctor. But that kind of switch isn't always possible; and patients always deserve the best I have to give them, even if I'm not the best doctor for their case. What, then, could I have done?

Perhaps we could have explicitly discussed the subtext of Aaron's accusations; I could have discussed race and explored why Aaron thought we were treating his family differently. I don't know if any of that would have been welcome: I don't think it's fair to ask anyone to have that conversation during the worst night of their lives. I do know that I was in no way equipped with the training or capacity to have that discussion at the time.

But something I could have done—something nobody did—is say, "I'm so very sorry for your loss" or "I wish there was another way" (see Chapter 4). I could have sat down. I could have offered tissues. I could have called the hospital pastor. It probably would have helped to do those things—to be humans, together.

I didn't do any of those things, largely because I had so little understanding of what was going on in that room. I didn't know the weight of the experiences that Janina and Aaron had brought to that room. I also didn't realize what I had brought to that room, what I was so uncomfortably folding and unfolding along with that pill packet: the implicit, unseen assumptions about Janina's care; about Aaron's investment in the pregnancy; about the homes they came from; about the future they had to offer children; about the care they had the right to expect.

To change those assumptions is going to take hard and constant work. To counter implicit bias requires all medical providers to question our motives, everywhere, to continually ask: "Is this what I should be doing? Do I know that's what she wants? Is that what I would offer a white woman or an older woman or a thinner woman?" This work requires an unyielding vigilance about—and sometimes against—our own brains.

For doctors like me, with years of training of that brain, with a pride in our cerebral aspect, treating our own thoughts as suspect can be a difficult task to accept. It is hard to be asked to fight with the part of ourselves that we are proudest of, that we have trained to be our livelihood and identity. But it's the only way forward.

.   .   .

I NEVER SAW Aaron or Janina again. I have always assumed that
this story represents the worst day of their lives, at least until then.
I have also assumed that when Aaron tells the story of this day, it
is full of the anger that he felt, anger of a man who knew—knew
from everything in his whole life—that we didn't value his children
or his feelings. That's fair. The way he experienced this day probably matches his experience as a black person in the United States:
devalued, disparaged, dismissed. I don't think we did anything to
convince either of them that something different was happening. I
don't think they're wrong.

But Janina left our care healthy and alive. She wasn't Violet. It
is such a very basic achievement that it doesn't warrant celebration.
Her life is the very least of what she deserved, coming out of our
care, the lowest of low bars.

And yet, let me recognize this: we could have done better; but
we have all too frequently, and all too recently, done much worse.
And so, around me and within me, I see change starting to happen:
not because it's easy, but because staying as we are is impossible.

Conclusion

Let's Go Home

It's the end of the workday on the second Wednesday of the month, which means I'm not going home. I'm on call tonight at the hospital. And I won't lie: I dread being on call. It's anxiety provoking and fatigue inducing to the point of nausea. There's a loneliness, a desperation, an exhaustion borne of being, it sometimes feels, the only one awake in the whole world.

But I also love being on call. There's a definitiveness to those dark hours, an energy. The patient needs care; the work must be done. We are the ones who have to do the work and make the hard decisions in the dark, through the night, until the morning. We have to figure it out; so we do. In some ways, being on call is when I'm the best doctor I can be. It's when I am in the fullest possession of whatever superpowers I have.

As we come to the end of this book, I want you to walk with me through a night on the labor and delivery floor, in real time. It is a night that is typical of my work: routine and amazing, everyday and earth-shattering, all at once.

This particular Wednesday, I walk onto the labor floor at 5:05 p.m., 5 minutes late, directly from a busy day at the clinic. My hands are clutching a takeout food container, betraying what I spent that 5 minutes doing. I'm still in my office clothes; but I'm here, as is the other attending doctor. We are the night team attendings, the bosses until the morning.

The other attending physician and I stand by the giant white-board that serves as the nerve center of our unit. The tired day attendings have gathered and are ready to hand over the care of all the patients. We divvy up the list. I take all the complicated patients, because I'm an MFM specialist, and that's my job. But I also snag an uncomplicated patient or two so the numbers won't be lopsided.

In room 1 is Ashlynn Jeffries, 38 years old with chronic hypertension and three prior cesarean deliveries, now 36 weeks pregnant. She was sent in from clinic with very high blood pressure values. As a patient with chronic hypertension, she is at risk for preeclampsia, but because of that same chronic high blood pressure, it can be difficult to tell when she's getting the disease. This is always really tricky. After half an hour or so in the hospital, her blood pressure has calmed down; all her labs have just returned and are normal.

At this moment, Ashlynn doesn't meet the criteria for pre-eclampsia with severe features; she may have preeclampsia or just her chronic hypertension, but either of those conditions would get delivered at 37 weeks. About an hour ago, the day team de-escalated and stopped her magnesium with the idea that she could be transferred off of L&D.

"Great," I say. "I'll stop by shortly to clear her for transfer."

"Yeah," says my colleague, "except that her nurse has just told me that Ashlynn has a headache."

A headache can be minor, but here it could change everything. A persistent headache can be a severe feature of preeclampsia, and if it lasts, it means that the plan needs to be changed from watching her to moving toward delivery. I ask the residents to go check Ashlynn out, offer her some acetaminophen, and recheck her blood pressure. We continue down the board.

In room 3 is Mina Kaye, a young, healthy woman 8 days past her due date who came in with her water broken. She really wanted a natural childbirth and progressed over the last 12 hours to 4 centimeters dilation. She's exhausted now, though, and her nurse stops by to tell us that she's starting to talk about requesting a cesarean delivery, even though she's not yet in active labor. The fetal heart tracing looked a little peaked a few minutes ago; it's improved now, but room 3 will be my first stop.

In room 7 is Susannah Roa, a patient with an autoimmune disease who is 27 weeks pregnant. The autoimmune disease has been quiet, but this morning, Susannah fell down three stairs on the way to her laundry room, hitting her belly. Traumas like this are worrisome not only for direct injury to Susannah herself but also, more insidiously, for their potential to cause a placental abruption. Even if the fall doesn't directly impact the placenta, shearing forces from the abrupt hit can cause the placenta to bleed and separate from the uterine wall. Susannah has no contractions, but she's very tender all over her abdomen, which is worrisome. Her labs are pending, and regardless, our pregnancy trauma protocol is for 24 hours of monitoring after any abdominal impact, so we make the decision to move her into the recovery room, for patients who can be monitored but are unlikely to deliver. That will free up a delivery room, although it's not as private or nice a place to spend the night. We'll check her out again once her lab results are available.

Ellen Danchev has just rolled into room 4; I'm told that she's having her second baby, at term. She came in with contractions; her cervix is dilated at 5 centimeters, she wants an epidural, and fetus is in vertex presentation (head down) on ultrasound. In other words: she is essentially uncomplicated. I look up at her tracing, which looks great. I tell the residents to call anesthesia; if she wants an epidural, they should get started on that now and not wait for me. I'll meet her when she's more comfortable.

That's the end of my portion of L&D, though my partner, the other attending on call with me, has just as many patients. It's a busy floor to walk into, but nothing extraordinary right now: nobody critically ill; no patients currently in the ICU; nobody at a periviable gestational age with terrible decisions to make, at least not yet. Just an ordinary night so far.

As I step back from the board, there's a resident standing at my shoulder, anxious to tell me about someone downstairs. The patient, Mercy David, had a cesarean delivery early in the morning, an emergent cesarean for a fetal heart rate that went down and didn't come up. Mercy's surgery was complicated by uterine atony: her uterus wouldn't contract after the delivery. The operating team had gotten the bleeding under control and documented the bleeding for the surgery as 1.5 liters, about 50 percent higher than for an average cesarean delivery. Because the team was worried about the bleeding, they instructed the day team to draw labs a few hours after surgery. That blood count returned with a very low hematocrit of 21, which they had expected to drop even further as time passed and her system equilibrated. Maybe she had lost 2 liters or more during the surgery; intraoperative estimation of blood loss is an imperfect art.

After that hematocrit was noted in the morning, Mercy was transfused 2 units of blood starting at 10 a.m. and finishing up around 4 p.m. Posttransfusion, labs were sent again, and that's why the resident is vibrating at my side. The posttransfusion hematocrit didn't go up: it's lower, at 20. That's not right. Where did those 2 units of blood that she received go? She's either still equilibrating or she's still bleeding, possibly internally. I ask the resident to go evaluate the patient—physical exam, vital signs, urine output—and check a stat repeat hematocrit. I need to hear about her within an hour, I say. If she doesn't look absolutely perfect, tell me sooner.

It's now almost 5:30 p.m., and I'm not even dressed yet. We say goodbye to the day team; they walk toward the door, rumpled and relaxed. I run upstairs, change into scrubs, and shovel two bites of the salad from my takeout container into my mouth while I push my feet into my battered clogs. I check my phone; the kids have been picked up, everybody is okay, spouse is almost home and will be in time to make sure the babysitter leaves before 6. I text back with my love and head back to labor and delivery.

I head right to room 3 to meet Mina. The room is dark and tense. Soothing music is playing, but Mina is in tears; her mother is leaning over her, rubbing her back, also in tears. It's been a long night followed by a long day, and Mina feels she can't do it any longer.

"Can't I just have a cesarean delivery?" she asks. "Please?"

"You can," I say, "if that's what you really want. But a cesarean isn't the cure for pain. It's a big surgery with a difficult recovery and usually involves a lot more pain. I'm pretty sure it's not the right first choice here. Can we try something else? Can we try to treat your pain and see how you feel? What are your thoughts about an epidural? I think it might mean you get a break and even some sleep."

Mina, it turns out, is terrified of needles. She relaxes a bit once she finds out that the epidural needle doesn't stay in your back; it's replaced by a slender and flexible catheter. Mina agrees to have the anesthesiologist come in to discuss the procedure. Now that she's no longer sobbing and her breathing has calmed down, the fetal heart tracing looks better. I ask the front desk to page anesthesia to room 3; they'll be here in a few minutes because they're just finishing up the epidural in room 4.

As I exit room 3, the nurse for room 1 calls me over: Ashlynn's headache is now a bit worse, not better, despite the acetaminophen. Her blood pressure is still normal, for now. I walk into the room and introduce myself. Ashlynn mentions that she's had rare migraines in her prepregnant life. Perhaps this is one? Ashlynn hedges; it's hard for her to remember if this feels different from her migraines. I review Ashlynn's labs: normal, without even protein in her urine sample, which is typical for preeclampsia. I talk with her: I'm worried in the context of her earlier blood pressure readings because it's not at all clear that this headache is a migraine and because it's getting worse. We make a plan to try one tablet of a stronger medication, which should knock out a migraine. If that doesn't work, we need to think that this headache is a new and severe sign of preeclampsia, and that would mean delivery. Ashlynn has just met me, and we're already in the middle of a 180-degree turn in her care from the de-escalation earlier in the afternoon. I am prepared for a longer conversation, but Ashlynn had been through something similar with her other kids, so she just nods, picks up her phone, and starts calling her family.

I stop by room 4. Ellen Danchev is immediately postepidural and still feeling her contractions, though she tells me that the pain is much better. I review her history and do a quick physical exam. I lay hands on her belly and estimate that she's having a good-sized baby, probably somewhere around 4 kilograms. I ask her if she's had diabetes screening during this pregnancy; Ellen laughs because I'm the third or fourth person to ask her this. She says that she was negative for diabetes, and in any case, her first baby was even bigger, so she's not worried. "I'm so glad to hear that," I say. "We tend to grow the right size fetuses for our bodies. If you're not worried, I'm not worried either." I write a quick note about her admission to the hospital and sign the resident's note.

I'm just thinking I'll get a few more bites of my dinner when the charge nurse tugs my arm. She's got a clipboard, and she's got a problem. On the schedule are three patients with scheduled inductions for this evening, scheduled to arrive at 7, 8, and 9 p.m. Two of them are already here, though it's barely 7 p.m. All our labor rooms are already full, and triage has several likely admissions. The charge nurse asks me what we're going to do, since we won't be able to accommodate these inductions in a timely fashion. They all need plans.

I review the charts quickly with a resident as I walk to triage. We reschedule two and admit one to the postpartum ward—Melanie Zientek—who is serious enough to need to be here for whenever a labor room frees up. All three patients, including Melanie, are very, very angry at this change of plans; this is understandable, but not easy. These discussions take a long time before they are willing to move forward.

While I'm at the triage desk finishing up the paperwork from these rescheduled patients, a patient rolls in on an ambulance stretcher, accompanied by paramedics. She is screaming that she has to push. The triage doctor is busy, and I'm right here, so I start talking to her, getting her history while I put on gloves. We wheel her into a curtained alcove—no beds available—and I examine her on the gurney. She's right: she's fully dilated and the fetal head is at +2 station. I grab a clean pair of gloves and start to put them on as I walk with the stretcher and the paramedics to the small operating room we keep as an overflow labor and delivery room for just such situations. As I walk, the patient tells me between panting breaths that her name is Blanca Castro, that she had two vaginal deliveries and then a prior cesarean in her last pregnancy for breech. She wanted a trial of labor this pregnancy. It turns out that Blanca was here earlier today with some intermittent contractions, but wasn't dilated at all. The nurse appears at the overflow room door, and together we bring Blanca into the room and help her transfer into the delivery bed. The paramedics wheel the gurney away, and we start to bustle around getting ready for delivery.

While the nurse is attaching Blanca's fetal monitor and her hospital bracelet, a resident taps me on the shoulder, and I meet her at the doorway, gloves still on. She tells me that Ashlynn's blood pressure is up, as high as 180, and her headache is persistent. "Well," I say, "at least she's declared herself." Now it's an easy diagnosis: preeclampsia with severe features, at 36 weeks. She needs to deliver.

And now, with these blood pressure values, Ashlynn is critically ill. The resident has given some medications urgently to keep her blood pressure from being high enough to be dangerous. If uncontrolled, blood pressure that high can lead to strokes or other serious complications. The resident tells me that Ashlynn's blood pressure is beginning to respond to medication, at least in the last 5 minutes, though it is still too high. I ask the resident to restart her magnesium, resend labs, and start working with anesthesia to stabilize her and prep her for the operating room. We will start Ashlynn's fourth cesarean delivery as soon as her blood pressure is stable.

I go back to Blanca, who is pushing beautifully. She delivers within 20 minutes; it's a rosy girl with lovely black hair. We deliver the placenta, and there's no need for any repair. The charge nurse tells me she will move Blanca to the PACU for recovery, though that's less private. But we need to clean this little overflow room as soon as possible, since we never know when we'll need it again. Blanca, holding her newborn, says she doesn't mind; she's so happy to have had the TOLAC she wanted. I run back to Ashlynn's room.

A resident stops me in the hallway. The postoperative patient downstairs, Mercy, has results from her hematocrit. Thankfully, it's a much more reasonable 25.2. That earlier value must have been taken too soon after the transfusion. The resident presents her full evaluation to me: no obvious bleeding, stable vital signs, satisfactory urine output; her abdominal exam is soft, not worrisome for internal bleeding. He tells me that the patient looks and feels pretty good, so we schedule her for a repeat lab in the very early hours of the morning and leave her alone.

As I stand there talking to him, I'm handed a sheet of lab results by a nurse. They belong to the 27-weeker with the abdominal trauma, Susannah. They're mostly reassuring, except that her fibrinogen, a blood-clotting protein, is strangely low. That result could be a sign of a large abruption. The story doesn't really fit, as she feels well aside from the aches and pains from the actual fall. No vaginal bleeding, no contractions, and the baby looks great. Placental abruptions can be tricky and hidden, though, so I decide to resend the labs 3 hours after the first ones and watch her closely. I wasn't going to give her steroids for fetal lung maturity, since her risk of delivery seemed so low. But this strange result changes my mind, so I go into the room to discuss steroids with her. I will still be very surprised if this develops into anything, I tell her, but we know that we're not always good at predicting who will need these. And at 27 weeks, antenatal corticosteroids can help a baby born prematurely live and be healthier than otherwise. Susannah agrees to the steroid shots, and the nurse goes off to collect her supplies.

Mina's nurse is calling. Mina is comfortable overall, postepidural, and got some much needed rest. She woke up after about a 45-minute nap and is feeling some pelvic pressure. I examine her, and hurray! She has gone from 4 centimeters to 9 centimeters, with a baby that is quite low and almost ready to be born. A little bit more time to become fully dilated, and she'll be ready to push.

I make it back to Ashlynn's room; the anesthesiologist and obstetrics resident are already there. Ashlynn's blood pressure has spiked again, despite that first dose of intravenous medication, and they're stroke-level again. We all agree that it's not safe to take her to the operating room until we stabilize her. The obstetrics resident is working her way down the emergent blood pressure protocol. "I was just about to call you," the resident says. "I'm maxed out on labetalol." That is, Ashlynn's already gotten the maximum dose of one of our first-line meds. As per the protocol for severe hypertension, we switch to a second med. That works much better; within 5 minutes of one dose of this second medication, Ashlynn's blood pressure calms down to 150s/100s. That's exactly where we want it: still high, but not dangerous. Now that she's in better control, it's the right time to take her for her surgery. She's still critically ill; but now we have the time we need to deliver her and get her better.

Serendipitously, the operating room is ready, anesthesia is ready, nursing is ready, the resident who will serve as surgical assist is ready, and I am ready. The anesthesia team start to roll her into the operating room to place the spinal for the cesarean, and Ashlynn's husband follows in the paper scrubs that dads wear in the operating room, the ones that make everyone look like a giant blue teddy bear. The second-year resident who will be my surgical assist goes in with them; she'll call for me once the spinal anesthesia is placed.

Mina's nurse is calling out: a lot of urgency to push in room 3. Do we need an epidural bolus for better anesthesia? No, Mina is fully dilated and the fetal head is so low, really ready. I think about calling the other attending for this delivery because I will need to get to the operating room in about 15 minutes. But Mina is very motivated after her short nap; she pushes with great energy. Only 10 minutes later, it's a boy! The new grandmother is in the corner, actually jumping up and down with joy. I deliver the placenta and do a very quick and simple repair of a first-degree tear. I say congratulations and run out because the spinal has just been placed in the operating room, and they're ready for me to start.

On the way to the operating room, the night chief resident stops me to tell me that there are three new admissions in triage. All three are close to term: two patients in labor and one who isn't but has poorly controlled diabetes and needs to be hospitalized for glucose control. "Perfect," I say. "Once we do this cesarean, we'll move Ashlynn to the PACU. And then we should have three rooms for the new patients. Right? Right. And don't forget Melanie Zientek—she shouldn't wait."

As we walk to the operating room, I ask the chief resident to bring me info on the diabetic patient while I'm operating: labs, finger sticks, doses of insulin, everything I need to know how critical her sugars are before we can even figure out where she goes. Does she need an ICU bed or to stay on labor and delivery rather than going to our less monitored antepartum unit? The chief will get back to me.

The rest of the night is a blur. Ashlynn's cesarean takes a while, as a fourth cesarean surgery generally does because of prior scarring. It is ultimately an uncomplicated surgery with a beautiful baby who, because of breathing problems likely related to his prematurity, is taken immediately by the pediatricians to the NICU. Ashlynn is sad while we finish her surgery, though we keep saying that the baby should do well, such mild prematurity, so close to term. It still feels bad that the baby is not in the room with us.

My partner attended Ellen Danchev's delivery while I was in the OR. Big baby—it turns out to have been bigger than we thought at 4.2 kilograms (9-plus pounds)—but uncomplicated. Ellen was right.

The patient with diabetes is, in the end, not that sick. I arrange her insulin and admission to the regular antepartum floor while suturing Ashlynn's uterus closed, and afterward I run to meet her and admit her and write notes. Then there are those admissions from triage, first one more for each attending and then two for each attending. Susannah, the patient with the weird fibrinogen, has repeat labs with a continuing low fibrinogen, but stable from prior and no other signs. We continue to watch her, and she continues to do absolutely nothing else concerning.

I run almost flat-out from room to room until about 4:45 a.m., when I tell the residents that I am going to rest, just for 15 minutes. They immediately recognize this for the lie that it is and tell me to relax; they'll just call me if they need me. When I get upstairs, I know that I'm tired, so I clip my pager to my collar so that I'll hear it and move the room's phone to the desk near my ear so I won't miss anything.

I sleep for an hour until I'm paged by an outpatient with a non-emergent issue. Groggily, I call down to the floor and get updates on everyone. The chief resident tells me that everything is under control, so I go back to sleep for another fitful half hour. I brush my teeth and come back down to L&D at 6:15 a.m., check on my remaining labor floor patients, and write updates for their charts. At some point, enough people delivered and transferred to postpartum that the charge nurse was able to send for Melanie Zientek; she's newly ensconced in a room and flashes me a confused look. She doesn't recognize me from earlier, when she was so upset at me. I reintroduce myself, write a note about her evening, and order her oxytocin infusion to start. In the PACU, Susannah is sleeping; she has a final set of labs scheduled for 10 a.m. If those are stable and she continues to look good, we can leave her alone until her 24 hours of monitoring are up.

Separated from Susannah by a striped curtain in the PACU, Ashlynn is in her postoperative stretcher, talking on her phone in a low voice. Her blood pressure is still high, but not stroke range, and she hasn't required any further treatment since her delivery.

And so, at this last round of the night, we again have nobody critically ill, critically preterm, or in the ICU. If you don't count the new babies, it looks like we're back to where we started the shift, though nobody can see how much work it took to get there.

At 7 a.m., I run down to the cafeteria as it opens and get a greasy egg on a bagel and a lukewarm coffee; it is simultaneously disgusting and heavenly. By 7:30 a.m., the morning residents arrive, and I sit in resident sign-out with both the night and day resident teams.

I spend about 10 minutes teaching about diabetes management in pregnancy, using our overnight admission as a teaching case. At 7:35 a.m., midsentence, my phone buzzes, and I look over. My husband is texting me that the big kids got on the bus to school and that he remembered to send the field trip permission slip with the eldest. I text back a thumbs-up emoji and keep talking about durations of action for different insulin types.

At 7:50 a.m., the night residents are gone and the new residents have dispersed to start working. I am waiting for the day attendings. I feel as if I've always been waiting for the day attendings. In these last few minutes of my overnight shift, I feel nauseated and hopeless. I feel that I have been working forever, that I will be working forever, that the day team of attendings will never come, and that I will never see sunshine again.

And then, at 8:03 a.m., they appear, all three of them at once. At the sight of them I become cheerful, even giddy. Morning has broken, and I can go home.

Our night team gathers at the board and signs out our patients to the day team, reversing the procedure from the night before. Nobody critically ill, nobody in the ICU, nobody extremely preterm in labor: all in all, a busy night, but not extraordinary in any medical way, except of course to the people who lived and bled and birthed through it.

I go to the call room to change back into my street clothes. I throw out my uneaten salad. By 8:40 a.m., I have left the hospital. I drive home, slowly and carefully. At home, I unpack my on-call bag. I shower. And then I crash in my bed and sleep very, very hard. After I wake up, I find an enormous bruise on my left leg; I don't know how or when during the night I got it, which seems about right.

I wake up slowly. I am getting dressed, making myself coffee, just enjoying being at home a few hours alone before I go to run errands or the kids get home from school. Once I have my coffee made, I sit down at the dining room table and log in to the hospital system. I just left them a few hours ago, but still: I want to know. What was Mercy's morning hematocrit? Did Ashlynn get sicker or continue to get better? How is her baby doing in the NICU? Did Susannah's labs get better, or did her condition worsen?

These patients were and are my sacred responsibility, and I want to make sure I did right by them; that I made choices and helped them make choices that set them on the right path. But more than that, my work gives me a front-row seat to the most interesting and compelling parts of human experience. And I still—always—want to know how these stories, these most important stories, end—and how, at the very same time, a new story begins.

Acknowledgments

This book would not be possible without the women who trust me with their care. Thank you for letting me be part of this work.

Thanks to my agent, Jessica Papin, who decided, immediately, that this book should become real, and who, with deep kindness, helped make it so. Thank you to my editor, Katie Adams at Liveright/Norton, who very intelligently not only knows how to edit a book, but how to teach a first-time author how to write one on the way. Thank you to my in-house editors, Marie Pantojan and Gina Iaquinta, who both jumped into this project with enthusiasm, and brought their significant smarts and expertise to bear.

Thank you to my amazing sisters, Shuli Karkowsky and Malki Karkowsky, two of my first readers and support staff and cheerleaders and general proof that sisters make the world go round.

Thank you to the rest of my first readers and navigators, including Emily Michaelson, Alison Spodek, Miriam Udel, Claire Sufrin, Ilana Kurshan, Jess Fechtor, and Mara Benjamin—you were reading me and providing hours of excellent judgment on these words well before they saw the light of day.

I want to thank all the people who provided expert review of various chapters to make sure I didn't say anything too wrong; any residual mistakes are my own. Many of these people are friends as well as doctors or academics (or both) and some of the busiest people in the world. Thank you, then, to Lisa Simmonds Rabinowitz, Shirlee Jaffe Lipshitz, Andrea Fick Greiner, Hayley Faith Solomon, Tracy Lee, Stacy Strehlow, Lisa Levy Zuckerwise, Maryann Long, Lisa Nathan, Ndaya Muleba, Emanuel D'Harcourt, Katherine Lin, Michael Reddy-Miller, and Rebecca Anhang Price. I also have to thank the academic corner of women's history of medicine, who gave graciously of their time and energy, including the incomparable Debby Levine, but also Sharrona Pearl, Jacqueline Antonovich, and the writers of Nursing Clio as well as Shannon Withycombe. Thank you to Yovanna Madhere and Faye Yvette McQueen for bringing their insights and experience to bear on a particularly tough chapter.

A huge thank you to the general cheerleaders and overall excellent support folks, including Rabbi Danya Ruttenberg for rabbinic/Twitter/gender language support. In this era of social media, I also want to thank two closed social media groups I belong to for being supportive, smart, and always awake.

Thank you to Gillian Steinberg, without whose coaching and critical thinking I would never have gotten the book proposal done, much less the book. I am not sure how anyone writes without her.

I want to thank my mom, Nancy Karkowsky, from whom I think I inherit any artistic talent I may have, and who has been doing PR for this book long before it went to press. I also want to thank my dad, Avi Karkowsky *z"l*, who always thought I'd make a great doctor. We miss him terribly.

Thank you to my kids. They helped make me into the person who could and would write this book. Additionally, they tolerated significant absences from Mama while I pursued this dream. For my eldest, who was extremely worried about my deadline, and kept asking how close I was: We made it!

And finally: thank you to my sweetie, Josh. I couldn't do this— any of this—without you. Miraculously, you have always and unwaveringly, from the first moment, maintained that all the things I have to say and feel are worth paying attention to. You maintain this even, and perhaps especially, when I'm convinced otherwise. Your love is a blessing in this and other ways.

Notes

CHAPTER 1: NAUSEA AND VOMITING OF PREGNANCY

1. Margie Profet, "Pregnancy Sickness as Adaptation: A Deterrent to Maternal Ingestion of Teratogens," in *The Adapted Mind: Evolutionary Psychology and the Generation of Culture*, ed. Jerome H. Barkow, Leda Cosmides, and John Tooby (New York: Oxford University Press, 1995), 327–61.

2. N. K. Kuşcu and F. Koyuncu, "Hyperemesis Gravidarum: Current Concepts and Management," *Postgraduate Medical Journal* 78, no. 916 (February 1, 2002): 76–79. https://doi.org/10.1136/pmj.78.916.76.

3. Committee on Practice Bulletins-Obstetrics. "ACOG Practice Bulletin No. 189: Nausea and Vomiting of Pregnancy," *Obstetrics & Gynecology* 131, no. 1 (2018): e15–30. https://doi.org/10.1097/AOG.0000000000002456.

4. J. A. Fitzgerald, "Death of Elderly Primigravida in Early Pregnancy. Charlotte Brontë," *New York State Journal of Medicine* 79, no. 5 (April 1979): 796–99; G. Weiss, "The Death of Charlotte Brontë," *Obstetrics & Gynecology* 78, no. 4 (October 1991): 705–8.

5. Fleetwood Churchill, *The Diseases of Females: Including Those of Pregnancy and Childbed* (Philadelphia: Lea and Blanchard, 1847), 387.

6. Churchill, *The Diseases of Females*, footnote, 381.

7. Churchill, *The Diseases of Females*, 387.

8. Shari Munch, "Chicken or the Egg? The Biological–Psychological Controversy

Surrounding Hyperemesis Gravidarum," *Social Science & Medicine* 55, no. 7 (2002): 1267–78.

9. E. Schjøtt-Rivers, "Hyperemesis Gravidarum: Clinical and Biochemical Investigations," *Acta Obstetricia et Gynecologica Scandinavica* 18, no. s1 (January 1938): 1–248. https://doi.org/10.3109/00016343809154869.

10. Schjøtt-Rivers, 19.

11. Denys V. I. Fairweather, "Nausea and Vomiting in Pregnancy," *American Journal of Obstetrics & Gynecology* 102, no. 1 (September 1, 1968): 135. https://doi.org/10.1016/0002-9378(68)90445-6.

12. Shari Munch, "Women's Experiences with a Pregnancy Complication: Causal Explanations of Hyperemesis Gravidarum," *Social Work in Health Care* 36, no. 1 (November 12, 2002): 59–75. https://doi.org/10.1300/J010v36n01_05.

13. "Practice Bulletin No. 52 Nausea & Vomiting of Pregnancy," April 2004, reaffirmed 2013. Replaced by Practice Bulletin No. 153, *Obstetrics & Gynecology* 126, no. 3 (September 2015): e1 –24.

14. Munch, "Chicken or the Egg?" 1269.

15. Munch, "Women's Experiences with a Pregnancy Complication," 59–75.

16. William A. Harvey and Mary Jane Sherfey, "Vomiting in Pregnancy: A Psychiatric Study," *Psychosomatic Medicine* 16, no. 1 (January 1954): 1–9.

17. Schjøtt-Rivers, "Hyperemesis Gravidarum," 18.

18. Schjøtt-Rivers, "Hyperemesis Gravidarum," 16.

19. Munch, "Chicken or the Egg?" 1267–78.

CHAPTER 2: CHOOSING A PROVIDER

1. Benjamin Gesundheit, Nachman Ash, Shraga Blazer, and Avraham I. Rivkind, "Medical Care for Terrorists—To Treat or Not to Treat?" *American Journal of Bioethics* 9, no. 10 (October 13, 2009): 40–42. https://doi.org/10.1080/15265160902985035; Nicki Pesik, Mark E. Keim, and Kenneth V. Iserson, "Terrorism and the Ethics of Emergency Medical Care." *Annals of Emergency Medicine* 37, no. 6 (June 1, 2001): 642–46. https://doi.org/10.1067/mem.2001.114316.

CHAPTER 3: GENETIC TESTING

1. Committee on Practice Bulletins, "Practice Bulletin No. 163 Summary: Screening for Fetal Aneuploidy," *Obstetrics & Gynecology* 127, no. 5 (May 2016): 979–81. https://doi.org/10.1097/AOG.0000000000001439.

2. "Practice Bulletin No. 162 Summary: Prenatal Diagnostic Testing for Genetic Disorders." *Obstetrics and Gynecology* 127, no. 5 (May 2016): 976–78. https://doi.org/10.1097/AOG.0000000000001438.

3. R. G. Resta, "Changing Demographics of Advanced Maternal Age (AMA) and the Impact on the Predicted Incidence of Down Syndrome in the United States: Implications for Prenatal Screening and Genetic Counseling," *American Journal of Medical Genetics Part A* 133A, no. 1 (2005): 31–36. Accessed February 6, 2018. http://onlinelibrary.wiley.com.elibrary.einstein.yu.edu/woll/doi/10.1002/ajmg.a.30553/full.

4. I. R. Merkatz, H. M. Nitowsky, J. N. Macri, and W. E. Johnson. "An Association between Low Maternal Serum Alpha-Fetoprotein and Fetal Chromosomal Abnormalities," *American Journal of Obstetrics & Gynecology* 148, no. 7 (April 1, 1984): 886–94.

5. Fergal D. Malone, Robert H. Ball, David A. Nyberg, Christine H. Comstock, George R. Saade, Richard L. Berkowitz, Susan J. Gross, et al., "First-Trimester Septated Cystic Hygroma: Prevalence, Natural History, and Pediatric Outcome," *Obstetrics & Gynecology* 106, no. 2 (August 2005): 288–94. https://doi.org/10.1097/01.AOG.0000173318.54978.1f.

6. This is the absolute most bonkers part of this. Why can't we use DNA from actual whole fetal cells in the maternal circulation? Then we could save time and get a whole chromosome or even a whole genome at once. It's not because there aren't enough of those cells—it's because there are too many of them, for too long. Those fetal cells can stick around for a long time—days, months, years. If I test a cell floating around, it may be from a last miscarriage or even a prior full-term pregnancy and not reflect the current pregnancy's genetics at all. In fact, there are male cells in the blood of women who carried a male pregnancy 25 years or so ago; women may die with cells from their sons and daughters somewhere inside them. In science, an organism that carries genetic material from other non-self organisms is considered a chimera. Thus, mothers, all of us, exhibit some level of chimerism. The chimera, of course, in Greek mythology, is a legendary monster composed of terrifying parts of multiple animals, often seen as the body of a lion, the head of a goat, and the tail of a snake, though other combinations have been described. I think this found metaphor about motherhood is almost too perfect.

7. "Committee Opinion No. 640: Cell-Free DNA Screening for Fetal Aneuploidy," *Obstetrics & Gynecology* 126, no. 3 (September 2015): e31–37.

8. "Trisomy 13," Genetics Home Reference. Accessed February 8, 2018. https://ghr.nlm.nih.gov/condition/trisomy-13.

CHAPTER 4: ANATOMY ULTRASOUND

1. Steven R. Lindheim, Stephanie Welsh, Nan Jiang, Amanda Hawkins, Lisa Kellar, Rose A. Maxwell, and Leah D. Whigham, "Trends in Management of Overweight and Obesity in Obstetrics & Gynecology, Family Medicine and Pediatrics 2011–15," *Journal of Obesity & Eating Disorders* 3, no. 1 (2017). https://doi.org/10.21767/2471-8203.100030.

2. Ann McNamara and Deborah Levine, "Intraabdominal Fetal Echogenic Masses: A Practical Guide to Diagnosis and Management," *RadioGraphics* 25, no. 3 (May 1, 2005): 633–45. https://doi.org/10.1148/rg.253045124.

3. From "Surgery—CraniotomyBurr Hole (Medical Transcription Sample Report)." Accessed February 25, 2018. http://www.mtsamples.com/site/pages/sample.asp?Type=85- . . . &Sample=176-Craniotomy%20-%20Burr%20Hole.

4. From "The Summer Day" in Mary Oliver, *New and Selected Poems*, vol. 1 (Boston: Beacon Press, 2004).

5. Susan Shepard, "A Fatal Case of Miscommunication," *Today's Hospitalist* (blog), May 9, 2012. https://www.todayshospitalist.com/a-fatal-case-of-miscommunication/.

6. Karen Davies, "The Body and Doing Gender: The Relations between Doctors and Nurses in Hospital Work," *Sociology of Health & Illness* 25, no. 7 (November 3, 2003): 720–42. https://doi.org/10.1046/j.1467-9566.2003.00367.x.

7. Orla T. Muldoon, and Jacqueline Reilly, "Career Choice in Nursing Students: Gendered Constructs as Psychological Barriers," *Journal of Advanced Nursing* 43, no. 1 (July 2003): 93–100. https://doi.org/10.1046/j.1365-2648.2003.02676.x.

8. Davies, "The Body and Doing Gender," 720–42.

9. Bobbi J. Carothers and Harry T. Reis, "Men and Women Are from Earth: Examining the Latent Structure of Gender," *Journal of Personality and Social Psychology* 104, no. 2 (February 2013): 385–407. https://doi.org/10.1037/a0030437.

10. "Men Are from ~~Mars~~ Earth, Women Are from ~~Venus~~ Earth," ScienceDaily. Accessed April 15, 2018. https://www.sciencedaily.com/releases/2013/02/130204094518.htm.

11. D'Ann Campbell, *Women at War with America: Private Lives in a Patriotic Era* (Cambridge, MA: Harvard University Press, 1984).

12. "2017 Data Brief Update: Current Trends of Men in Nursing—Center for Interdisciplinary Health Workforce Studies | Montana State University." Accessed April 20, 2018. http://healthworkforcestudies.com/publications-data/data_brief_update_current_trends_of_men_in_nursing.html; U.S. Census Bureau, "Male Nurses Becoming More Commonplace, Census Bureau Reports." The U. S. Census Bureau, February 25, 2013. Accessed April 20, 2018. https://www.census.gov/newsroom/press-releases/2013/cb13-32.html.

13. Eliza Lo Chin, "Looking Back over the History of Women in Medicine," MomMD. Accessed April 20, 2018. https://www.mommd.com/lookingback .shtml; "More Women Than Men Enrolled in U.S. Medical Schools in 2017." Accessed May 5, 2019. https://news.aamc.org/press-releases/article/applicant -enrollment-2017/; Paul Jolly, "Medical Education in the United States, 1960–1987," *Health Affairs* 7, suppl. 2 (January 1988): 144–57. https://doi .org/10.1377/hlthaff.7.2.144.

14. David Hughes, "When Nurse Knows Best: Some Aspects of Nurse/Doctor Interaction in a Casualty Department," *Sociology of Health & Illness* 10, no. 1 (March 1, 1988): 1–22. https://doi.org/10.1111/1467-9566.ep11340102.

15. M. Leonard,S. Graham, and D. Bonacum, "The Human Factor: The Critical Importance of Effective Teamwork and Communication in Providing Safe Care." *Quality and Safety in Health Care* 13, suppl 1 (October 1, 2004): i85–90. https://doi.org/10.1136/qshc.2004.010033.

16. R. Morgan and C. Westmoreland, "Survey of Junior Hospital Doctors' Attitudes to Cardiopulmonary Resuscitation," *Postgraduate Medical Journal* 78, no. 921 (July 1, 2002): 413–15. https://doi.org/10.1136/pmj.78.921.413.

CHAPTER 5: PERIVIABLE BIRTH

1. "NICHD Neonatal Research Network (NRN): Extremely Preterm Birth Outcome Data." NIH. Accessed January 20, 2019. https://www1.nichd.nih.gov/ epbo-calculator/Pages/epbo_case.aspx.

CHAPTER 6: TRIAL OF LABOR AFTER CESAREAN

1. Bruce Cohen and Meredith Atkins, "Brief History of Vaginal Birth after Cesarean Section," *Clinical Obstetrics and Gynecology* 44, no. 3 (September 2001): 604. https://journals.lww.com/clinicalobgyn/Citation/2001/09000/Brief_History_ of_Vaginal_Birth_After_Cesarean.17.aspx.

2. Emma L. Barber, Lisbet S. Lundsberg, Kathleen Belanger, Christian M. Pettker, Edmund F. Funai, and Jessica L. Illuzzi, "Indications Contributing to the Increasing Cesarean Delivery Rate," *Obstetrics & Gynecology* 118, no. 1 (July 2011): 29–38. https://doi.org/10.1097/AOG.0b013e31821e5f65.

3. ACOG, "Safe Prevention of the Primary Cesarean Delivery," Obstetric Care Consensus No. 1, March 2014. Accessed November 27, 2017. https://www.acog .org/Resources-And-Publications/Obstetric-Care-Consensus-Series/Safe -Prevention-of-the-Primary-Cesarean-Delivery.

4. T. S. Nesbitt, J. E. Scherger, and J. L. Tanji, "The Impact of Obstetrical Liability on Access to Perinatal Care in the Rural United States," *Journal of Rural Health* 5, no. 4 (October 1989): 321–35.

5. Sindhu K.Srinivas, Dylan S. Small, Michelle Macheras, Jesse Y. Hsu, Donna Caldwell, and Scott Lorch, "Evaluating the Impact of the Laborist Model of Obstetric Care on Maternal and Neonatal Outcomes," *American Journal of Obstetrics & Gynecology* 215, no. 6 (December 1, 2016): 770.e1–770.e9. https://doi.org/10.1016/j.ajog.2016.08.007.

6. Cohen and Atkins, "Brief History of Vaginal Birth after Cesarean Section," 604.

7. ACOG Committee on Obstetric Practice, "Committee Opinion #266: Placenta Accreta," *Obstetrics & Gynecology* 99, no. 1 (January 1, 2002): 169–70. https://doi.org/10.1016/S0029-7844(01)01748-3.

8. ACOG Committee on Obstetric Practice. "Committee Opinion #266: Placenta Accreta," 169–70; "Obstetric Care Consensus No. 7: Placenta Accreta Spectrum." *Obstetrics and Gynecology* 132, no. 6 (December 2018): e259–75. https://doi.org/10.1097/AOG.0000000000002983.

9. ACOG, "ACOG Practice Bulletin No. 115: Vaginal Birth after Previous Cesarean Delivery." *Obstetrics & Gynecology* 116, no. 2 Pt 1 (August 2010): 450–63. https://doi.org/10.1097/AOG.0b013e3181eeb251.

10. David J.Birnbach, Brenda A. Bucklin, and Franklin Dexter, "Impact of Anesthesiologists on the Incidence of Vaginal Birth after Cesarean in the United States: Role of Anesthesia Availability, Productivity, Guidelines, and Patient Safety," *Seminars in Perinatology* 34, no. 5 (October 2010): 318–24.

11. Richard G. Roberts, Mark Deutchman, Valerie J. King, George E. Fryer, and Thomas J. Miyoshi, "Changing Policies on Vaginal Birth after Cesarean: Impact on Access," *Birth* 34, no. 4 (December 1, 2007): 316–22. https://doi.org/10.1111/j.1523-536X.2007.00190.x.

12. Marian MacDorman, Eugene Declercq, and Fay Menacker, "Recent Trends and Patterns in Cesarean and Vaginal Birth after Cesarean (VBAC) Deliveries in the United States," *Clinics in Perinatology* 38, no. 2 (June 1, 2011): 179–92. https://doi.org/10.1016/j.clp.2011.03.007.

13. M. G. Pinette, J. Kahn, K. L. Gross, J. R. Wax, J. Blackstone, and A. Cartin, "Vaginal Birth after Cesarean Rates Are Declining Rapidly in the Rural State of Maine," *Journal of Maternal-Fetal & Neonatal Medicine* 16, no. 1 (July 2004): 37–43. https://doi.org/10.1080/14767050412331831111.

14. Committee on Practice Bulletins-Obstetrics, "Practice Bulletin No. 184: Vaginal Birth after Cesarean Delivery," *Obstetrics & Gynecology* 130, no. 5 (2017): e217–33. https://doi.org/10.1097/AOG.0000000000002398.

15. ACOG, "ACOG Committee Opinion No. 560: Medically Indicated Late-Preterm and Early-Term Deliveries," *Obstetrics & Gynecology* 121, no. 4 (April 2013): 908–10. https://doi.org/10.1097/01.AOG.0000428648.75548.00.

16. Paula M. Lantz, Lisa Kane Low, Sanjani Varkey, and Robyn L. Watson, "Doulas as Childbirth Paraprofessionals: Results from a National Survey," *Women's Health Issues* 15, no. 3 (May 2005): 109–16. https://doi.org/10.1016/j .whi.2005.01.002; Amy Moffat, "The Labor of Labour Support: How Doulas Negotiate Care Work" (PhD thesis, University of California, Merced, 2014).

CHAPTER 7: STILLBIRTH

1. "ACOG Practice Bulletin No. 102: Management of Stillbirth," *Obstetrics & Gynecology* 113, no. 3 (March 2009): 748–61. https://doi.org/10.1097/AOG .0b013e31819e9ee2.

2. Joanne Cacciatore, Ingela Rådestad, and J. Frederik Frøen, "Effects of Contact with Stillborn Babies on Maternal Anxiety and Depression," *Birth* 35, no. 4 (2008): 313–20. https://doi.org/10.1111/j.1523-536X.2008.00258.x.

3. R. Smith, K. Maiti, and R. J. Aitken, "Unexplained Antepartum Stillbirth: A Consequence of Placental Aging?" *Placenta* 34, no. 4 (April 2013): 310–13. https://doi.org/10.1016/j.placenta.2013.01.015.

4. "Clinical Management Guidelines for Obstetrician-Gynecologists Number 45, August 2003: (Replaces Committee Opinion Number 152, March 1995)," *Obstetrics & Gynecology* 102, no. 2 (August 2003): 417–27. https://doi.org/10 .1097/00006250-200308000-00045.

5. The efficacy of continuous fetal monitoring has not been proved, but almost all delivery setups, including home delivery, offer some level of intermittent fetal monitoring during labor, though often analog (auscultative) methods may be utilized. See Valerie Smith, Cecily M. Begley, Mike Clarke, and Declan Devane, "Professionals' Views of Fetal Monitoring during Labour: A Systematic Review and Thematic Analysis," *BMC Pregnancy and Childbirth* 12 (December 27, 2012): 166. https://doi.org/10.1186/1471-2393-12-166.

6. GBD 2015 Child Mortality Collaborators, "Global, Regional, National, and Selected Subnational Levels of Stillbirths, Neonatal, Infant, and Under-5 Mortality, 1980–2015: A Systematic Analysis for the Global Burden of Disease Study 2015," *The Lancet* 388, no. 10053 (October 8, 2016): 1725–74. https://doi .org/10.1016/S0140-6736(16)31575-6.

7. The GRIT Study Group, "A Randomised Trial of Timed Delivery for the Compromised Preterm Fetus: Short Term Outcomes and Bayesian Interpre-

tation," *British Journal of Obstetrics and Gynaecology* 110 (January 2003): 27–32. Accessed July 9, 2018. https://obgyn.onlinelibrary.wiley.com/doi/epdf/10.1046/j.1471-0528.2003.02014.x.

CHAPTER 8: INFORMED CONSENT

1. Committee on Practice Bulletins—Obstetrics, "ACOG Practice Bulletin No. 154: Operative Vaginal Delivery," *Obstetrics & Gynecology* 126, no. 5 (November 2015): e56–65. https://doi.org/10.1097/AOG.0000000000001147.
2. Herbert B. Peterson, Zhisen Xia, Joyce M. Hughes, Lynne S. Wilcox, Lisa Ratliff Tylor, and James Trussell, "The Risk of Ectopic Pregnancy after Tubal Sterilization," *The New England Journal of Medicine* 336, no. 11 (March 13, 1997): 762–67. https://doi.org/10.1056/NEJM199703133361104.
3. "The Little-Known History of the Forced Sterilization of Native American Women," *JSTOR Daily*, August 25, 2016. https://daily.jstor.org/the-little-known-history-of-the-forced-sterilization-of-native-american-women/.
4. P. R. Reilly, "Involuntary Sterilization in the United States: A Surgical Solution," *The Quarterly Review of Biology* 62, no. 2 (June 1987): 153–70.
5. "Births Financed by Medicaid," *The Henry J. Kaiser Family Foundation* (blog), October 13, 2016. https://www.kff.org/medicaid/state-indicator/births-financed-by-medicaid/.
6. Tubal reconstructive surgery is possible, though isn't always successful. Alternatively, IVF can be used: it doesn't require tubes because the fertilization happens in the lab. However, many insurance companies won't pay for either of these options if the reason for tubal infertility is a prior sterilization. You have to be sure.
7. There are institutions that will allow the tubal to be performed, though in this situation the hospital cannot be reimbursed. This creates a solution where the patient gets what they need, but this is, of course, not sustainable financially for hospitals. It also creates a concern for medicolegal liability, with improperly completed paperwork, so some hospitals cannot routinely pursue this course of action.
8. Sonya Borrero, Nikki Zite, Joseph E. Potter, James Trussell, and Kenneth Smith, "Potential Unintended Pregnancies Averted and Cost Savings Associated with a Revised Medicaid Sterilization Policy," *Contraception* 88, no. 6 (December 2013): 691–96. https://doi.org/10.1016/j.contraception.2013.08.004.
9. Andrea Ries Thurman and Torri Janecek, "One-Year Follow-up of Women with Unfulfilled Postpartum Sterilization Requests," *Obstetrics & Gyne-*

cology 116, no. 5 (November 2010): 1071–77. https://doi.org/10.1097/AOG .0b013e3181f73eaa.

10. Kiera Butler, "The Scary Truth about Childbirth," *Mother Jones,* January/ February 2017. Accessed June 15, 2018. https://www.motherjones.com/ politics/2017/01/childbirth-injuries-prolapse-cesarean-section-natural -childbirth/; "Giving Birth Made Me Question the Informed Consent Process during Childbirth," Self (website). Accessed June 10, 2018. https://www.self .com/story/informed-consent-in-childbirth.

11. "Giving Birth Made Me Question the Informed Consent Process during Childbirth."

12. This is the preferred nomenclature, as per activists within the fat acceptance community; see https://www.naafaonline.com/dev2/about/index.html.

13. Ibrahim A. Hammad, Suneet P. Chauhan, Everett F. Magann, and Alfred Z. Abuhamad, "Peripartum Complications with Cesarean Delivery: A Review of Maternal-Fetal Medicine Units Network Publications," *Journal of Maternal-Fetal & Neonatal Medicine* 27, no. 5 (March 1, 2014): 463–74. https://doi.org/10 .3109/14767058.2013.818970.

14. Lovina Machado, "Emergency Peripartum Hysterectomy: Incidence, Indications, Risk Factors and Outcome," *North American Journal of Medical Sciences* 3, no. 8 (August 2011): 358–61. https://doi.org/10.4297/najms.2011.358.

15. ACOG Committee on Ethics, "ACOG Committee Opinion No. 439: Informed Consent," *Obstetrics & Gynecology* 114, no. 2 Pt. 1 (August 2009): 401–8. https://doi.org/10.1097/AOG.0b013e3181b48f7f.

CHAPTER 9: MEDICAL SYSTEMS AND HOME BIRTH

1. Patrick T. O'Gara, Frederick G. Kushner, Deborah D. Ascheim, Donald E. Casey, Mina K. Chung, James A. de Lemos, Steven M. Ettinger, et al., "2013 ACCF/AHA Guideline for the Management of ST-Elevation Myocardial Infarction: A Report of the American College of Cardiology Foundation/American Heart Association Task Force on Practice Guidelines," *Journal of the American College of Cardiology* 61, no. 4 (January 29, 2013): e78–140. https://doi.org/10.1016/j.jacc.2012.11.019.

2. Committee on Practice Bulletins—Obstetrics, ACOG, "Practice Bulletin No. 130: Prediction and Prevention of Preterm Birth," *Obstetrics & Gynecology* 120, no. 4 (October 2012): 964–73. https://doi.org/10.1097/AOG.0b013e3182723b1b.

3. For how this situation arose via a complicated series of decisions by the FDA regarding this drug, as well as contemporaneous problems with compounded

medications (the closest less expensive alternative), read Yesha Patel and Martha M. Rumore, "Hydroxyprogesterone Caproate Injection (Makena) One Year Later," *Pharmacy and Therapeutics* 37, no. 7 (July 2012): 405–11; and "Oversight Improves after Contaminated Compounded Drugs Killed Dozens, but Risks Remain." Accessed August 8, 2018. http://pew.org/2ndGxil.

4. Anne Rossier Markus, Ellie Andres, Kristina D. West, Nicole Garro, and Cynthia Pellegrini, "Medicaid Covered Births, 2008 through 2010, in the Context of the Implementation of Health Reform." *Women's Health Issues* 23, no. 5 (September 1, 2013): e273–80. https://doi.org/10.1016/j.whi.2013.06.006; "Births Financed by Medicaid." *The Henry J. Kaiser Family Foundation* (blog), October 13, 2016. https://www.kff.org/medicaid/state-indicator/births-financed-by -medicaid/.

5. Paul J. Meis, Mark Klebanoff, Elizabeth Thom, Mitchell P. Dombrowski, Baha Sibai, Atef H. Moawad, Catherine Y. Spong, et al, "Prevention of Recurrent Preterm Delivery by 17 Alpha-Hydroxyprogesterone Caproate." *The New England Journal of Medicine* 348, no. 24 (June 12, 2003): 2379–85. https://doi .org/10.1056/NEJMoa035140.

6. Not the smartphone mini-application kind of widget. The economics basic-unit-of-production kind of widget; see: "Widget (Economics)," *Wikipedia*, February 11, 2018. https://en.wikipedia.org/w/index.php?title=Widget_ (economics)&oldid=825119151.

7. Tim Harford, "The Steel Box That Changed Global Trade," *BBC News*, January 9, 2017, sec. Business. https://www.bbc.co.uk/news/business-38305512.

8. T. J. Mathews, Marian F. MacDorman, and Fay Menacker, "Infant Mortality Statistics from the 1999 Period Linked Birth/Infant Death Data Set," *National Vital Statistics Reports* 50, no. 4 (January 30, 2002): 1–28. From the Centers for Disease Control and Prevention, National Center for Health Statistics, National Vital Statistics System. https://www.cdc.gov/nchs/pressroom/02facts/99infant .htm.

9. "Reducing Early Elective Deliveries Webinar." Pdf. Accessed July 23, 2018. https:// innovation.cms.gov/Files/transcripts/StrongStart_ElectiveDelivery_Trscrpt.pdf.

10. Daniel J. Riskin, Thomas C. Tsai, Loren Riskin, Tina Hernandez-Boussard, Maryanne Purtill, Paul M. Maggio, David A. Spain, and Susan I. Brundage, "Massive Transfusion Protocols: The Role of Aggressive Resuscitation Versus Product Ratio in Mortality Reduction," *Journal of the American College of Surgeons* 209, no. 2 (August 1, 2009): 198–205. https://doi.org/10.1016/j .jamcollsurg.2009.04.016. Many maternal outcomes for patients receiving MTP

have been proven to be improved compared with hemorrhaging patients who do not receive MTP; however, the reduction in maternal mortality is difficult to prove given that, thankfully, maternal death is a rare outcome. I am thus extrapolating from other proven maternal outcomes, as well as from the literature in war trauma in the nonpregnant population. See Molly Lepic, Danielle M. Greer, Jessica J. F. Kram, Niraj Nijhawan, and Andra Cicero, "Use of Massive Transfusion Protocol: Maternal Outcomes in Patients with Severe Obstetric Hemorrhage [22K]," *Obstetrics & Gynecology* 131 (May 2018): 124S–25S. https://doi.org/10.1097/01.AOG.0000533524.00973.3c.

11. *"Marcus Welby, M.D."* *Wikipedia*, June 6, 2018. https://en.wikipedia.org/w/index.php?title=Marcus_Welby,_M.D.&oldid=844639230.

12. This section relies heavily on this excellent book: Judith Walzer Leavitt, *Brought to Bed: Childbearing in America, 1750–1950*, 30th Anniversary Edition (New York: Oxford University Press, 2016).

13. Leavitt, *Brought to Bed*, 27.

14. Frances E. Kobrin, "The American Midwife Controversy: A Crisis of Professionalization," *Bulletin of the History of Medicine* 40, no. 4 (1966): 350–63.

15. Abraham Flexner, "Medical Education in the United States and Canada." A report to the Carnegie Foundation for the Advancement of Teaching. Bulletin Number 4 (1910). http://www.columbia.edu/itc/hs/pubhealth/rosner/p8773/readings/flexner1.pdf.

16. Leavitt, *Brought to Bed*, 189.

17. Leavitt, *Brought to Bed*, 184.

18. Leavitt, *Brought to Bed*, 199.

19. Leavitt, *Brought to Bed*, 203.

20. Leavitt, *Brought to Bed*, 203.

21. Leavitt, *Brought to Bed*, 208.

22. Leavitt, *Brought to Bed*, 205.

23. "The Mistrust of Science." Pdf. Commencement Speech by Dr. Atul Gawande to the California Institute of Technology, June 2016. Accessed August 10, 2018. http://www.todroberts.com/USF/Mistrust_of_Science.pdf.

24. Joseph R. Wax, F. Lee Lucas, Maryanne Lamont, Michael G. Pinette, Angelina Cartin, and Jacquelyn Blackstone, "Maternal and Newborn Outcomes in Planned Home Birth vs Planned Hospital Births: A Meta-Analysis," *American Journal of Obstetrics & Gynecology* 203, no. 3 (September 2010): 243.e1–243.e8. https://doi.org/10.1016/j.ajog.2010.05.028.

25. ACOG Committee on Obstetric Practice, "ACOG Committee Opinion

No. 476: Planned Home Birth," *Obstetrics & Gynecology* 117, no. 2 Pt 1 (February 2011): 425–28. https://doi.org/10.1097/AOG.0b013e31820eee20.

26. Melissa Cheyney, Marit Bovbjerg, Courtney Everson, Wendy Gordon, Darcy Hannibal, and Saraswathi Vedam, "Outcomes of Care for 16,924 Planned Home Births in the United States: The Midwives Alliance of North America Statistics Project, 2004 to 2009," *Journal of Midwifery & Women's Health*, January 30, 2014, Wiley Online Library. Accessed August 10, 2018. https://onlinelibrary.wiley.com/doi/full/10.1111/jmwh.12172; Robyn M. Kennare, Marc J. N. C. Keirse, Graeme R. Tucker, and Annabelle C. Chan, "Planned Home and Hospital Births in South Australia, 1991–2006: Differences in Outcomes," *The Medical Journal of Australia* 192, no. 2 (January 18, 2010): 76–80; Hilda Bastian, Marc J. N. C. Keirse, and Paul A. L. Lancaster, "Perinatal Death Associated with Planned Home Birth in Australia: Population Based Study," *British Medical Journal* 317, no. 7155 (August 8, 1998): 384–88.

27. Catherine Elton, "American Women: Birthing Babies at Home," *Time*, September 4, 2010. http://content.time.com/time/magazine/article/0,9171,2011940,00.html.

28. CNMs are amazing, and I have both enjoyed working extensively with them and learned a tremendous amount from them. CNMs undergo rigorous and validated training and enter the midwifery field with prior formal training in nursing (usually at least a master's degree). They are also licensed in all 50 states in the United States. A similar credential, certified midwife (CM), is now available in six states and represents very similar rigorous training; CMs must pass the same exams as CNMs, though they may not always have a prior degree in nursing. Both holders of the CM credential and holders of the CNM credential generally work with a doctor on some level (which varies by state) and are formally credentialed to provide independent prenatal, delivery, and postpartum care for a normal healthy pregnancy.

29. "State By State." Midwives Alliance of North America (website), October 17, 2013. https://mana.org/about-midwives/state-by-state.

30. Amy Tuteur, "Why Is American Home Birth So Dangerous?" Opinion, *The New York Times*, April 30, 2016. Accessed February 13, 2019. https://www.nytimes.com/2016/05/01/opinion/sunday/why-is-american-home-birth-so-dangerous.html.

31. Saraswathi Vedam, Kathrin Stoll, Marian MacDorman, Eugene Declercq, Renee Cramer, Melissa Cheyney, Timothy Fisher, Emma Butt, Y. Tony Yang, and Holly Powell Kennedy, "Mapping Integration of Midwives across the United States: Impact on Access, Equity, and Outcomes," *PLOS ONE* 13, no. 2 (February 21, 2018): e0192523. https://doi.org/10.1371/journal.pone.0192523.

32. Saraswathi Vedam, Lawrence Leeman, Melissa Cheyney, Timothy J. Fisher, Susan Myers, Lisa Kane Low, and Catherine Ruhl, "Transfer from Planned Home Birth to Hospital: Improving Interprofessional Collaboration," *Journal of Midwifery & Women's Health* 59, no. 6 (November 1, 2014): 624–34. https://doi.org/10.1111/jmwh.12251; Amelia Hill, "Home Birth: 'What the Hell Was I Thinking?'" *The Guardian*, April 15, 2011, sec. Life and style. http://www.theguardian.com/lifeandstyle/2011/apr/16/home-birth-trial-or-rewarding.

CHAPTER 10: MATERNAL MORTALITY AND
RACIAL DISPARITIES IN HEALTH CARE

1. Marian F. MacDorman, Eugene Declercq, Howard Cabral, and Christine Morton, "Recent Increases in the U.S. Maternal Mortality Rate: Disentangling Trends from Measurement Issues," *Obstetrics & Gynecology* 128, no. 3 (September 2016): 447–55. https://doi.org/10.1097/AOG.0000000000001556.
2. "Health Spending." OECD Data. Accessed September 16, 2018. http://data.oecd.org/healthres/health-spending.htm.
3. CDC, "Pregnancy Mortality Surveillance System | Maternal and Infant Health | CDC," January 16, 2019. https://www.cdc.gov/reproductivehealth/maternalinfanthealth/pregnancy-mortality-surveillance-system.htm.
4. CDC, "Pregnancy Mortality Surveillance System | Maternal and Infant Health."
5. CDC, "Pregnancy Mortality Surveillance System | Maternal and Infant Health"; Daniel B. Nelson, Michelle H. Moniz, and Matthew M. Davis, "Population-Level Factors Associated with Maternal Mortality in the United States, 1997–2012," *BMC Public Health* 18, no. 1 (August 13, 2018): 1007. https://doi.org/10.1186/s12889-018-5935-2.
6. Rebecca M. Puhl and Chelsea A. Heuer, "Obesity Stigma: Important Considerations for Public Health," *American Journal of Public Health* 100, no.6 (June 2010): 1019–1028. Accessed October 3, 2018. https://www.ncbi.nlm.nih.gov/pmc/articles/PMC2866597/.
7. Amy M. Kilbourne, Galen Switzer, Kelly Hyman, Megan Crowley-Matoka, and Michael J. Fine, "Advancing Health Disparities Research within the Health Care System: A Conceptual Framework," *American Journal of Public Health* 96, no. 12 (December 2006): 2113–21. https://doi.org/10.2105/AJPH.2005.077628.
8. Joses A. Jain, Lorene A. Temming, Mary E. D'Alton, Cynthia Gyamfi-Bannerman, Methodius Tuuli, Judette M. Louis, Sindhu K. Srinivas, et al., "SMFM Special Report: Putting the 'M' Back in MFM: Reducing Racial and Ethnic Disparities in Maternal Morbidity and Mortality: A Call to Action,"

American Journal of Obstetrics & Gynecology 218, no. 2 (February 2018): B9–17. https://doi.org/10.1016/j.ajog.2017.11.591.

9. Alan Nelson, "Unequal Treatment: Confronting Racial and Ethnic Disparities in Health Care," *Journal of the National Medical Association* 94, no. 8 (August 2002): 666–68.

10. Brian D. Smedley, Adrienne Y. Stith, and Alan R. Nelson, eds., *Unequal Treatment: Confronting Racial and Ethnic Disparities in Health Care (with CD)* (Washington, DC: National Academies Press, 2003). https://doi.org/10.17226/12875.

11. K. A. Schulman, J. A. Berlin, W. Harless, J. F. Kerner, S. Sistrunk, B. J. Gersh, R. Dubé, et al., "The Effect of Race and Sex on Physicians' Recommendations for Cardiac Catheterization," *The New England Journal of Medicine* 340, no. 8 (February 25, 1999): 618–26. https://doi.org/10.1056/NEJM199902253400806.

12. Keith Payne, Laura Niemi, and John M. Doris, "How to Think about 'Implicit Bias,'" *Scientific American*, March 27, 2018. Accessed September 12, 2018. https://www.scientificamerican.com/article/how-to-think-about-implicit-bias/; "Project Implicit." Accessed September 12, 2018. https://implicit.harvard.edu/implicit/. And the following article from 1998 is a classic: A. G. Greenwald, D. E. McGhee, and J. L. Schwartz. "Measuring Individual Differences in Implicit Cognition: The Implicit Association Test," *Journal of Personality and Social Psychology* 74, no. 6 (June 1998): 1464–80.

13. AAMC, "Diversity in the Physician Workforce: Facts and Figures 2014." Accessed September 23, 2018. https://www.aamc.org/data/workforce/reports/439214/workforcediversity.html; AAMC, "Section II: Current Status of the U.S. Physician Workforce," AAMC Interactive Report. Accessed September 23, 2018. http://www.aamcdiversityfactsandfigures.org/section-ii-current-status-of-us-physician-workforce/index.html.

14. U.S. Census Bureau, "QuickFacts: UNITED STATES." Accessed September 23, 2018. https://www.census.gov/quickfacts/fact/table/US/PST045217.

15. Jordan J. Cohen, Barbara A. Gabriel, and Charles Terrell, "The Case for Diversity in the Health Care Workforce," *Health Affairs* 21, no. 5 (September 1, 2002): 90–102. https://doi.org/10.1377/hlthaff.21.5.90.

16. Devah Pager, Bart Bonikowski, and Bruce Western, "Discrimination in a Low-Wage Labor Market: A Field Experiment," *American Sociological Review* 74, no. 5 (October 1, 2009): 777–99. https://doi.org/10.1177/000312240907400505.

17. Katherine L. Milkman, Modupe Akinola, and Dolly Chugh, "Temporal Distance and Discrimination: An Audit Study in Academia," *Psychological Science* 23, no. 7 (July 1, 2012): 710–17. https://doi.org/10.1177/0956797611434539.

Index

umbilical cord fluids, 149

uterine bleeding, 137–40

uterine rupture

danger of, 117–18

patient narrative of, 118–22

uteroplacental unit, 142–43, 149

vacuum deliveries

narrative, 157–63

as operative vaginal delivery, 157

vaginal birth after cesarean (VBAC).
See cesarean birth, trial of labor
after

vaginal deliveries, issue of consent for,
170–72

vaginal delivery, operative. See forceps
deliveries; vacuum deliveries

Valerie's story, 137–41, 152

verbal consent, 159–60, 163

Victoria's story, 13–18

Violet's story, 226–28

vomiting. See nausea and vomiting

water breaking, 178, 226–28

weight, as maternal risk factor, 141–42
See also obese patients

women's health, discussing, xv–xvii
See also reproductive life and health,
author on

Yvonne's story, vii–viii, xi, xiii–xv,
xx–xxi

zidovudine, 100